DASH DIET FOR HEALTHY COUPLE
COUPLE

Cookbook

More than 220 Recipes for Two to reduce triglycerides and cholesterol!
Delight Yourself and Your Partner with the Healthiest Dietary Approach Recipes!

BY
MICHELLE SANDLER

2 BOOKS IN 1

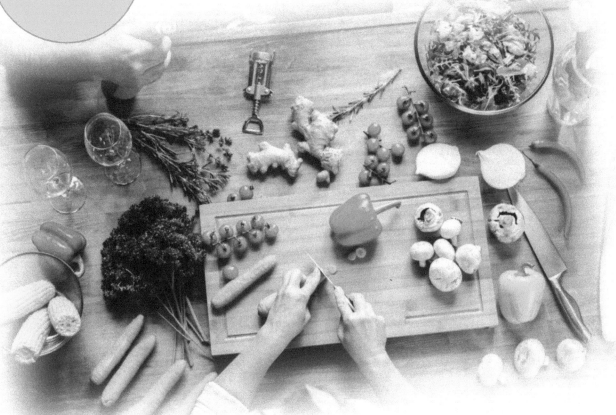

Table of Contents

Have you ever known the Dash Diet?

The DASH Diet is a fantastic dietary regimen specifically for **heart health**.

It is in fact one of the few diets in the world specifically designed to reduce triglycerides and bad cholesterol in the blood, in order to improve blood pressure and blood circulation.

The purpose of the DASH diet is therefore to improve the health of the person who follows it. After careful clinical studies conducted in the United States, the Dash Diet is currently recommended by many medical associations around the world, especially for people at risk of developing cardiovascular disease.

In the Dash Diet the word **DASH** is an acronym: it stands for *Dietary Approaches to Stop Hypertension.*

Dash Diet is not linked to weight loss. In fact, the number of calories introduced is equal to the daily nutritional requirements (it is a so-called isocaloric diet) and not less. However, there are some **variants of the Dash Diet** specific for overweight people, based on the consumption of the same foods but in smaller portions in order to reduce the calories acquired.

What are the additional benefits of following the DASH diet?

Clinical studies show that a high consumption of fruits and vegetables reduces the risk of developing **diabetes, cancer, atherosclerosis**, and other diseases typical of old age. Replacing saturated fats, found in butter or cheese, with unsaturated fats, found in nuts, olive oil, and seeds, helps reduce triglycerides and cholesterol, greatly reducing the chance of developing cardiovascular disease.

Anyone can follow the Dash Diet: **women**, **men**, **kids**, **older people**, **sedentary people** and **athletes**!

How many times did you go crazy to find two or three different recipes to cook for you and your partner or family?

I think all of us should follow this diet to have a much healthier lifestyle and live better and longer, and this is why I created this a fantastic book series about DASH Diet: *"Dash Diet for Couple Cookbook"* is the first collection of this series and it was born to give all my brilliant readers the possibility to stop going crazy to find the right recipes for all family members! Indeed, *"Dash Diet for Couple"* is the collection of 2 of my best books: *"The Dash Diet for Him Cookbook"* and *"The Dash diet Her Cookbook"*. And, what is no better than more than 220 Dash recipes for a couple of persons who want to increase their heart health and prevent diseases!

Dash Diet involves eating certain foods and reducing (or sometimes eliminating) others.

Yes foods:

- Vegetables
- Carbohydrates from whole grains
- Fruit
- Low-fat dairy products
- Fish
- White meat
- Vegetable oils
- Sea Salt/Himalayan salt

No foods:

- Red meat
- Animal fats
- Sugar
- Alcohol
- Processed products
- Synthetic salt (sodium chloride)
- Preservatives

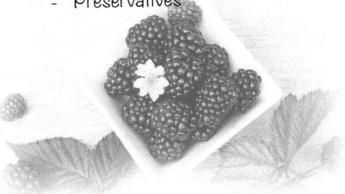

BOOK 1: DASH DIET FOR HER

CHAPTER 1. BREAKFAST AND SNACKS

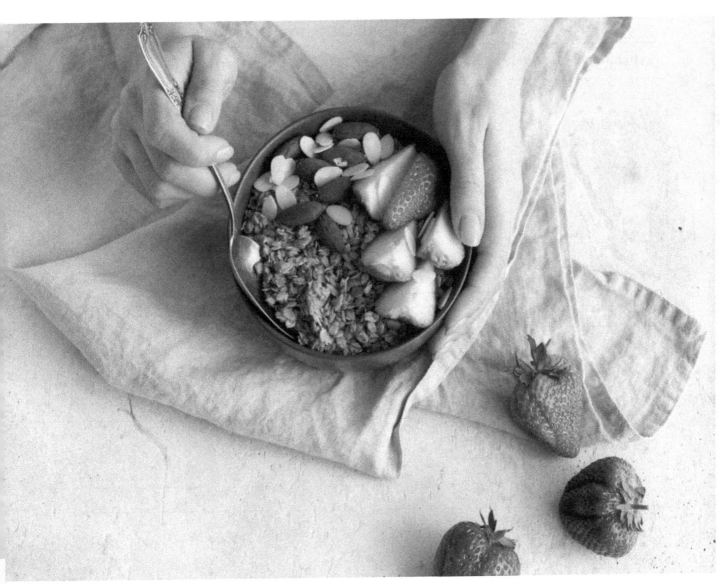

1) SHRIMP AND EGG MEDLEY

Preparation Time: 15 minutes	Cooking Time: Zero	Servings:

Ingredients:

- ✓ 4 hard-boiled eggs, shelled and chopped
- ✓ 1 pound cooked shrimp, shelled and seeded, chopped
- ✓ 1 sprig fresh dill, chopped

Ingredients:

- ✓ ¼ cup mayonnaise
- ✓ 1 teaspoon Dijon mustard
- ✓ 4 fresh lettuce leaves

Directions:

- ❖ Take a large bowl and add the ingredients listed (except the lettuce).

- ❖ Mix well.
- ❖ Serve over a topping of lettuce leaves. Enjoy!

2) ZUCCHINI OMELETTE WITH CHEESE

Preparation Time: 10 minutes	Cooking Time: 20 minutes	Servings: 3

Ingredients:

- ✓ 4 large eggs
- ✓ 2-3 medium zucchini

Ingredients:

- ✓ 1-2 garlic cloves, crushed
- ✓ 4 tablespoons grated cheese Season as needed

Directions:

- ❖ Take a bowl and add the grated zucchini, be sure to peel it because the skin is bitter.
- ❖ Take a bowl and add the eggs, crushed garlic and cheese.

- ❖ Pour the mixture into a hot pan with a little oil and put it on medium heat, keep a lid on it.
- ❖ Once the egg is well cooked, and the bottom is crispy and golden, serve and enjoy with a garnish of chopped parsley. Enjoy!

3) HEALTHY PEACH OATMEAL

Preparation Time: 10 minutes	Cooking Time: 10 minutes	Servings: 8

Ingredients:

- ✓ 4 cups old-fashioned rolled oats
- ✓ 3 ½ cups low-fat milk
- ✓ 3 ½ cups water 1 teaspoon cinnamon powder

Ingredients:

- ✓ 1/3 cup palm sugar
- ✓ 4 peaches, chopped

Directions:

- ❖ Add the oats, milk, cinnamon, water, sugar and peaches to your Robot.
- ❖ Stir well. Close the lid and cook for 10 minutes on high pressure.

- ❖ Release the pressure naturally over 10 minutes.
- ❖ Divide the mix into bowls and serve!

4) TRADITIONAL OMELETTE

Preparation Time: 10 minutes	**Cooking Time**: 5 minutes	**Servings**: 6

Ingredients:

- ✓ 2 tablespoons almond milk Just a pinch of pepper
- ✓ 6 eggs, broken and beaten
- ✓ 2 tablespoons parsley, chopped

Ingredients:

- ✓ 1 tablespoon low-fat cheese, shredded
- ✓ 1 cup water

Directions:

- ❖ Take a bowl and add the eggs, almond milk, pepper, cheese and parsley. Whisk well.
- ❖ Take a skillet that would fit in your robot and grease with cooking spray. Pour the egg mixture into the pan.

- ❖ Add one cup of water to the pan and place a steamer basket in it. Add the skillet to the basket.
- ❖ Close the lid and cook on HIGH pressure for 5 minutes. Release the pressure naturally on 10 minutes.
- ❖ Remove the lid and divide the omelet between serving plates. Enjoy!

5) TOMATO EGG PIE

Preparation Time: 10 minutes	**Cooking Time**: 5 minutes	**Servings**: 2

Ingredients:

- ✓ 2 whole eggs
- ✓ ½ cup fresh basil, chopped
- ✓ 2 tablespoons olive oil

Ingredients:

- ✓ ½ teaspoon red pepper flakes, crushed
- ✓ 1 cup grape tomatoes, chopped Salt and pepper to taste

Directions:

- ❖ Take a bowl and whisk in eggs, salt, pepper, red pepper flakes and mix well. Add the tomatoes, basil and stir.

- ❖ Take a skillet and place it over medium-high heat.
- ❖ Add the egg mixture and cook for 5 minutes until cooked and scrambled. Enjoy!

6) THYME WAFFLES WITH CHEESE

Preparation Time: 15 minutes	**Cooking Time**:	**Servings**: 2

Ingredients:

- ✓ ½ cup mozzarella cheese, finely shredded
- ✓ ¼ cup Parmesan cheese
- ✓ ¼ large cauliflower
- ✓ ½ cup collard greens
- ✓ 1 large egg
- ✓ 1 green onion stalk
- ✓ ½ tablespoon olive oil

Ingredients:

- ✓ ½ teaspoon garlic powder
- ✓ ¼ teaspoon salt
- ✓ ½ tablespoon sesame seeds
- ✓ 1 teaspoon fresh thyme, chopped
- ✓ ¼ teaspoon ground black pepper
- ✓

Directions:

- ❖ Place the cauliflower, cabbage tops, spring onion and thyme in a food processor and pulse until smooth.
- ❖ Distribute the mixture into a bowl and mix with the rest of the ingredients.
- ❖

- ❖ Heat a waffle iron and transfer the mixture evenly to the waffle iron.
- ❖ Cook until it forms a waffle and serve in a serving dish.

7) LEMON AND BLUEBERRY MUFFINS

Preparation Time: 5 minutes	**Cooking Time:** 25 minutes	**Servings: 12 muffins**

- ✓ 1 cup white whole wheat flour
- ✓ 1 cup all-purpose flour
- ✓ 2 teaspoons baking powder
- ✓ 1 teaspoon of baking soda
- ✓ ⅓ cup of granulated sugar
- ✓ Peel of 1 lemon, finely grated

- ✓ 1 cup of low-fat buttermilk
- ⅓ cup of canola oil
- ✓ 1 egg
- ✓ 1 teaspoon of vanilla extract
- ✓ 1½ cups fresh or frozen blueberries (not thawed)

❖ Preheat the oven to 400°F (205°C). Line a standard 12-cup muffin mold with paper liners or spray with nonstick cooking spray.

❖ In a medium bowl, combine the whole wheat and all-purpose flours, baking powder and baking soda.

❖ In a large bowl, combine the sugar, lemon zest, buttermilk, canola oil, egg and vanilla, and beat with an electric mixer on medium speed until well combined.

❖ Add the dry ingredients to the wet ingredients in two or three batches, whisking just to combine after each addition. Gently add the blueberries.

❖ Spoon the batter evenly into the prepared muffin cups. Bake in the preheated oven for 20-25 minutes, until the tops are golden brown and a toothpick inserted in the center comes out clean.

❖ Let the muffins cool in the pan for a few minutes, then transfer them to a wire rack. Serve warm or at room temperature.

8) MAPLE OATMEAL PANCAKES

Preparation Time: 15 minutes	**Cooking Time:** 15 minutes	**Servings:4**

- ✓ 1½ cups old-fashioned rolled oats
- ✓ ½ cup whole wheat flour
- ✓ 1 teaspoon ground cinnamon
- ✓ 1 teaspoon baking powder

- ✓ 2 cups of low-fat buttermilk
- ✓ 2 tablespoons of maple syrup
- ✓ 1 egg
- ✓ Kitchen spray

❖ In a medium bowl, combine the oats, flour, cinnamon and baking powder.

❖ In a large bowl, whisk together the buttermilk, maple syrup and egg.

❖ Add the dry mixture to the wet mixture in two or three batches, stirring well after each addition. Let stand for about 10 minutes, until the mixture becomes bubbly.

❖ Spray a nonstick skillet with cooking spray and heat over medium heat. For each pancake, use about ¼ cup of batter, and cook for 2 to 3 minutes, until bubbles appear on the surface. Flip and continue to cook for 1 to 2 minutes, until golden brown on the other side. Cook remaining batter in batches of three or four until done. Serve immediately.

9) ZUCCHINI FRITTERS WITH PUMPKIN SPICES

Preparation Time: 10 minutes	**Cooking Time:** 15 minutes	**Servings: 4**

Ingredients:

- ✓ 2 cups shredded zucchini
- ✓ 1¼ cup whole wheat flour
- ✓ 2 teaspoons baking powder
- ✓ 1 teaspoon pumpkin pie spice
- ✓ 2 eggs

Ingredients:

- ✓ 1 cup plus 2 tablespoons low-fat milk
- ✓ 2 tablespoons unsalted butter, melted
- ✓ 2 tablespoons of light brown sugar
- ✓ 1 teaspoon of vanilla extract
- ✓ Kitchen spray

Directions:

❖ Wrap the shredded zucchini in a clean dish towel and squeeze out as much water as possible.

❖ In a large bowl, combine the flour, baking powder, and pumpkin pie spice.

❖ In a medium bowl, whisk together the eggs, milk, butter, brown sugar and vanilla. Add the wet ingredients to the dry ingredients and whisk to combine. Stir in the zucchini.

❖ Spray a large nonstick skillet with cooking spray and heat over medium heat. For each pancake, use about ⅓ of batter (about 4 inches in diameter) and cook for 2 to 3 minutes, until bubbles appear on the surface. If the batter is too thick, add a splash of milk. Flip the pancakes and cook 1 to 2 minutes, until the other side is golden brown. Serve warm.

10) SPINACH AND EGG CHEESE PIE

Preparation Time: 5 minutes	**Cooking Time:** 20 minutes	**Servings: 4**

Ingredients:

- ✓ 10 ounces (283 g) of frozen chopped spinach, thawed and squeezed
- ✓ 4 eggs
- ✓ ¼ cup of chunky sauce

Ingredients:

- ✓ ¼ cup crumbled goat cheese
- ✓ Freshly ground pepper, to taste
- ✓ Kitchen spray

❖ Preheat oven to 325ºF (163ºC). Spray four 6-ounce / 170-g ramekins with cooking spray.

❖ For each ramekin, cover the bottom with spinach. Make a slight indentation in the center of the spinach and crack an egg.

❖ Add 1 tablespoon of sauce and 1 tablespoon of goat cheese to the egg. Sprinkle with pepper.

❖ Place the ramekins on a baking sheet and bake in the preheated oven for about 20 minutes, until the whites are completely set but the yolk is still a little runny. Serve immediately.

11) QUICK BREAKFAST BURRITOS

Preparation Time: 5 minutes	**Cooking Time:** 5 minutes	**Servings: 4**

Ingredients:

- ✓ 4 egg whites
- ✓ 2 eggs
- ✓ ¼ cup low-fat milk
- ✓ ⅛ teaspoon of freshly ground pepper
- ✓ 4 whole wheat tortillas

Ingredients:

- ✓ ½ cup (2 oz / 57 g) of low-fat sharp Cheddar cheese
- ✓ 1 cup canned black beans, rinsed and drained
- ✓ ¼ cup chopped shallots
- ✓ ½ cup of sauce
- ✓ ¼ cup non-fat sour cream

❖ In a microwaveable dish, whisk together the egg whites, eggs, milk and pepper. Cook the mixture in the microwave on high temperature for 3 minutes. Remove the dish from the microwave and stir. Cook in the microwave for 1 additional minute, or until the eggs are set.

❖ Place 1 tortilla on each of four microwave-safe plates. Divide the egg mixture evenly over the tortillas. Top each with a quarter of the cheese, beans and scallions.

❖ Wrap burritos and microwave for 30 seconds. Serve immediately, topped with salsa and sour cream.

12) ASPARAGUS TOAST WITH POACHED EGGS

Preparation Time: 5 minutes	**Cooking Time:** 15 minutes	**Servings: 4**

Ingredients:

- ✓ 4 slices of sourdough wholemeal bread
- ✓ 1-pound (454 g) asparagus, chopped
- ✓ 2 tablespoons of olive oil

Ingredients:

- ✓ ½ teaspoon of freshly ground pepper
- ✓ 8 eggs
- ✓ ¼ cup (about 1 ounce / 28 g) of grated Parmesan cheese

❖ Preheat the grill. Place a pot of water over medium-high heat and bring to a boil.

❖ Place the bread and asparagus on a large rimmed baking sheet, drizzle with the olive oil and sprinkle with pepper. Bake in the preheated oven for about 1 to 2 minutes, until the bread is toasted on top. Flip the bread over and bake for another 1 to 2 minutes, until the other side is toasted. Transfer the bread to four serving plates and place the asparagus back on the grill. Bake for 5-8 minutes, until tender.

❖ Meanwhile, with the water in the saucepan over low heat, carefully crack the eggs. Reduce the heat to medium-low and simmer for about 4 minutes, until the whites are set and the yolks are still runny.

❖ Arrange asparagus equally on toast. Add 2 eggs to each slice and sprinkle with cheese. Serve immediately.

13) SWEET POTATO HASH WITH BRUSSELS SPROUTS

Preparation Time: 5 minutes	**Cooking Time**: 20 minutes	**Servings**: 4

Ingredients:

- ✓ 2 tablespoons of olive oil
- ✓ 2 garlic cloves, minced
- ✓ ½ red onion, diced
- ✓ 2 sweet potatoes, peeled and diced

Ingredients:

- ✓ 8 ounces (227 g) Brussels sprouts, cut and sliced crosswise
- ✓ 1 teaspoon fresh chopped thyme
- ✓ ½ teaspoon of freshly ground pepper
- ✓ 4 eggs

Directions:

- ❖ Fill a medium saucepan with about 4 inches of water and bring to a boil over high heat.
- ❖ Meanwhile, heat the olive oil in a large skillet over medium heat. Add the garlic and cook, stirring, for 1 minute. Add the onion and cook, stirring occasionally, until it begins to soften, about 2 to 3 minutes.
- ❖ Increase the heat to medium-high and add the sweet potatoes. Cook, stirring occasionally, until the potatoes begin to brown, about 8 minutes.

- ❖ Add the Brussels sprouts and cook for 4 to 5 minutes, until they begin to brown. Season with thyme and pepper.
- ❖ When the water in the saucepan boils, carefully add the eggs. Reduce the heat to low and simmer for 6 minutes. Drain and rinse the eggs under cold water.
- ❖ Divide the hash evenly among four serving plates. Carefully peel the eggs and place one on each hash portion. Serve immediately.

14) QUICHE IN A MICROWAVEABLE CUP

Preparation Time: 2 minutes	**Cooking Time**: 3 minutes	**Servings**: 1

Ingredients:

- ✓ ½ cup chopped, thawed and drained frozen spinach (or ½ cup packaged fresh spinach)
- ✓ 1 large egg
- ✓ ⅓ cup of low-fat milk

Ingredients:

- ✓ 1 teaspoon of olive oil
- ✓ Freshly ground black pepper, to taste
- ✓ ½ slice of wholemeal bread, torn into small pieces

Directions:

- ❖ If using fresh spinach, place it in a cup with 2 tablespoons of water. Cover with a paper towel and cook in the microwave for 1 minute. Remove from the microwave and drain the water from the spinach before adding it back into the cup. If using frozen spinach, make sure it is completely thawed and drained.

- ❖ Crack the egg into the bowl with the spinach and add the milk, olive oil and pepper. Whisk until well mixed.
- ❖ Add the bread and mix gently, but do not whisk.
- ❖ Place the cup in the microwave and cook on high heat for 1 minute until the egg is cooked and the quiche is slightly puffy.
- ❖ Enjoy immediately.

15) AVOCADO AND EGG TOAST

Preparation Time: 5 minutes	**Cooking Time**: 5 minutes	**Servings**: 1

Ingredients:

- ✓ 2 eggs
- ✓ 2 slices of wholemeal bread
- ✓ 1 small avocado

Ingredients:

- ✓ 1 teaspoon of freshly squeezed lime juice
- ✓ Freshly ground black pepper, to taste

Directions:

- ❖ Toast the bread and cook the eggs according to your preference.
- ❖ Peel and mash the avocado with the lime juice and pepper.

- ❖ Spread the avocado evenly on each slice of toast, then top each slice with a fried egg.
- ❖ Serve immediately.

16) OATMEAL WITH ALMONDS AND BLUEBERRIES

Preparation Time: 10 minutes	**Cooking Time**: 17 minutes	**Servings**: 4

Ingredients:	Ingredients:
✓ 1 cup of skim or low-fat milk ✓ 1 cup of water ✓ 1 teaspoon ground cinnamon	✓ 1 cup steel cut oats ✓ 1 cup blueberries ✓ ½ cup sliced almonds

Directions:

❖ In a medium saucepan over medium heat, whisk together milk, water and cinnamon.

❖ When the mixture begins to boil, add the steel cut oats and bring to a boil.

❖ Reduce heat to low and simmer for 15 minutes.

❖ About 2 minutes before the end of cooking, add the blueberries and almonds and mix well.

❖ Serve immediately.

---

17) GREEN PEACH SMOOTHIE

Preparation Time: 5 minutes	**Cooking Time**: 0 minutes	**Servings**: 1

Ingredients:	Ingredients:
✓ 2 cups fresh spinach (or ⅓ cup frozen) ✓ 1 cup frozen peaches (or fresh, pitted) ✓ 1 cup of ice	✓ ½ cup of skim or low-fat milk ✓ ½ cup nonfat or low-fat Greek yogurt ✓ ½ teaspoon of vanilla extract ✓ Optional: no-calorie sweetener of your choice

Directions:

❖ Optional: no-calorie sweetener of your choice

❖ Optional: no-calorie sweetener of your choice

---

18) BANANA AND PEANUT BUTTER SMOOTHIE

Preparation Time: 5 minutes	**Cooking Time**: 0 minutes	**Servings**: 1

Ingredients:	Ingredients:
✓ 1 cup of skim or low-fat milk ✓ 1 cup of ice ✓ ¼ cup nonfat or low-fat Greek yogurt	✓ 1 frozen banana, cut into slices ✓ 1 tablespoon of peanut butter

Directions:

❖ Add all ingredients to a blender and process until smooth.

❖ Enjoy immediately.

19) EGG MUFFINS WITH BROCCOLI AND CHEESE

Preparation Time: 15 minutes	**Cooking Time**: 30 minutes	**Servings**: 4

Ingredients:

- ✓ 1 tablespoon of olive oil
- ✓ 1 small head of broccoli, cut into small florets (about 4 cups)
- ✓ 8 big eggs
- ✓ ¼ cup of skimmed milk
- ✓ 1 teaspoon of onion powder
- ✓ 1 teaspoon garlic powder

Ingredients:

- ✓ ¼ teaspoon of kosher salt or sea salt
- ✓ ½ teaspoon of ground black pepper
- ✓ ½ teaspoon dry mustard powder
- ✓ 1 cup shredded cheddar cheese, split
- ✓ Kitchen spray

Directions:

- ❖ Preheat the oven to 350°F (180°C).
- ❖ Heat the olive oil in a medium skillet over medium heat. Add broccoli and sauté 4 to 5 minutes, until soft.
- ❖ In a large bowl, whisk together the eggs, milk, onion powder, garlic powder, salt, black pepper and mustard powder. Add the sautéed broccoli and half of the Cheddar cheese.

- ❖ Coat a 12-cup muffin mold with cooking spray. Evenly distribute egg mixture into each cup. Sprinkle with remaining cheddar cheese. Bake for 18-22 minutes, until eggs are set.
- ❖ Let the muffins cool slightly before removing them from the pan.
- ❖ Place egg muffins in airtight microwave-safe containers and refrigerate for up to 5 days or freeze for up to 2 months. Reheat in microwave for 1 to 2 minutes on high speed, until heated through.

20) GREEK SCRAMBLED EGGS

Preparation Time: 10 minutes	**Cooking Time**: 10 minutes	**Servings**: 4

Ingredients:

- ✓ 1 tablespoon of olive oil
- ✓ 1 pint grape or cherry tomatoes, quartered
- ✓ 2 cups chopped cabbage
- ✓ 2 garlic cloves, peeled and chopped
- ✓ 8 big eggs

Ingredients:

- ✓ ¼ teaspoon of kosher salt or sea salt
- ✓ ¼ teaspoon ground black pepper
- ✓ ¼ cup of crumbled feta cheese
- ✓ ¼ cup chopped Italian flat leaf parsley

Directions:

- ❖ Heat olive oil in a large nonstick skillet over medium heat. Add the tomatoes and cabbage. Sauté for 2 to 3 minutes, until the cabbage and tomatoes are slightly soft. Add the garlic. Reduce the heat of the skillet to low.

- ❖ In a medium bowl, whisk together the eggs, salt and black pepper. Pour the egg mixture into the skillet, slowly folding the eggs in until foamy and scrambled. Remove from heat and add the feta and parsley.
- ❖ Store the scramble in airtight microwave-safe containers and refrigerate for up to 5 days. Heat in microwave on high speed for 60-90 seconds, until heated through.

CHAPTER 2. LUNCH

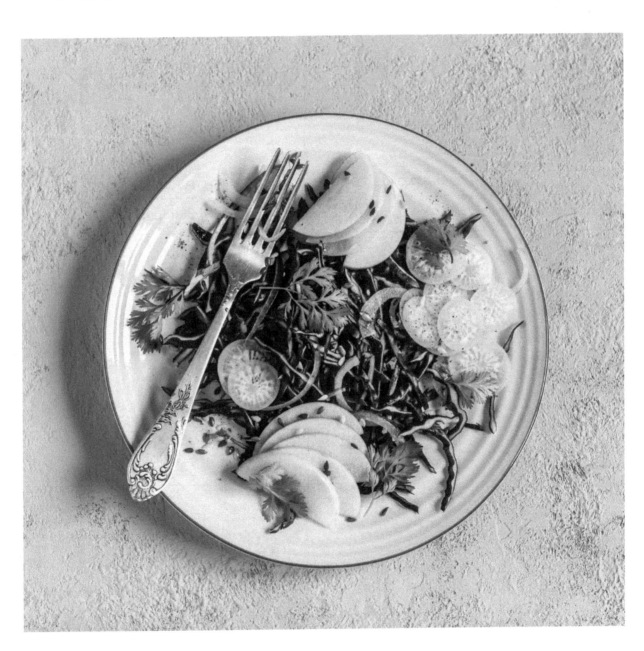

21) ROASTED RED POTATOES AND ASPARAGUS

Preparation Time:	Cooking Time:	Servings:

Ingredients:

- ✓ 1 1/2 pounds red potatoes, cut into chunks
- ✓ 2 tablespoons extra-virgin olive oil
- ✓ 12 garlic cloves, thinly sliced
- ✓ 1 tablespoon and 1 teaspoon dried rosemary

Ingredients:

- ✓ 4 teaspoons dried thyme
- ✓ 2 teaspoons sea salt
- ✓ 1 bunch fresh asparagus, trimmed and cut into 1-inch pieces

Directions:

- ❖ Preheat oven to 425 degrees F.
- ❖ In a baking dish, combine first 5 ingredients and 1/2 of the sea salt. Cover with aluminum foil.
- ❖ Bake 20 minutes in the oven. Combine the asparagus, oil, and salt. Cover, and bake for about 15 minutes, or until potatoes become tender.

- ❖ Increase oven temperature to 450 degrees F.
- ❖ Remove aluminum foil and bake for 8 minutes, until potatoes turn lightly browned.

22) ROASTED GREEN BEANS IN BUTTER WITH GARLIC AND LIME

Preparation Time:	Cooking Time:	Servings:

Ingredients:

- ✓ 1 1/2 pounds potatoes, cut into chunks
- ✓ 4 tablespoons butter
- ✓ 12 garlic cloves, thinly sliced

Ingredients:

- ✓ 2 tablespoons lime juice
- ✓ 2 teaspoons sea salt
- ✓ 1 bunch fresh green beans, trimmed and cut into 1-inch pieces

Directions:

- ❖ Preheat oven to 425 degrees F. In a baking dish, combine first 5 ingredients and 1/2 of the sea salt.
- ❖ Cover with aluminum foil. Bake 20 minutes in the oven. Combine the green beans, oil, and salt.

- ❖ Cover, and bake for about 15 minutes, or until potatoes become tender. Increase oven temperature to 450 degrees F.
- ❖ Remove aluminum foil and bake for 8 minutes, until potatoes turn lightly browned.

23) ROASTED ESCAROLE AND HEARTS OF PALM

Preparation Time:	Cooking Time:	Servings:

Ingredients:

- ✓ 1 1/2 pounds escarole, cut into chunks
- ✓ 3 tablespoons extra virgin olive oil
- ✓ 12 garlic cloves, thinly sliced

Ingredients:

- ✓ 1 tablespoon and 1 teaspoon dried rosemary
- ✓ 4 teaspoons dried thyme
- ✓ 2 teaspoons sea salt
- ✓ 1 bunch hearts of palm, trimmed and cut into 1-inch pieces

- ❖ Preheat oven to 425 degrees F. In a baking dish, combine first 5 ingredients and 1/2 of the sea salt.
- ❖ Cover with aluminum foil. Bake 20 minutes in the oven. Combine the hearts of palm, oil and salt.

- ❖ Cover and bake for about 15 minutes, or until escarole is tender. Increase oven temperature to 450 degrees F.
- ❖ Remove aluminum foil and bake for 8 minutes, until potatoes turn lightly browned.

24) ROASTED ITALIAN CABBAGE AND ASPARAGUS

Preparation Time:	Cooking Time:	Servings:

Ingredients:

- ✓ 1 1/2 pounds kohlrabi, chopped
- ✓ 2 tablespoons extra-virgin olive oil
- ✓ 12 garlic cloves, thinly sliced
- ✓ 1 tablespoon Italian seasoning

Ingredients:

- ✓ 4 teaspoons dried thyme
- ✓ 2 teaspoons sea salt
- ✓ 1 bunch fresh asparagus, trimmed and cut into 1-inch pieces

Directions:

- ❖ Preheat oven to 425 degrees F. In a baking dish, combine first 5 ingredients and 1/2 of the sea salt.
- ❖ Cover with aluminum foil. Bake 20 minutes in the oven.
- ❖ Combine the asparagus, oil and salt.

- ❖ Cover and bake for about 15 minutes, or until kohlrabi becomes tender. Increase oven temperature to 450 degrees F.
- ❖ Remove foil, and bake for 8 minutes, until kohlrabi becomes lightly browned.

25) ROASTED POTATOES AND SWEET POTATOES WITH WALNUTS

Preparation Time:	Cooking Time:	Servings:

Ingredients:

- ✓ 1/2 pound red potatoes, cut into chunks
- ✓ ½ pound sweet potatoes, cut into chunks
- ✓ 2 tablespoons peanut oil
- ✓ 12 garlic cloves, thinly sliced

Ingredients:

- ✓ 1 tablespoon and 1 teaspoon herbes de Provence
- ✓ 2 teaspoons sea salt
- ✓ 1 bunch fresh asparagus, trimmed and cut into 1-inch pieces

Directions:

- ❖ Preheat oven to 425 degrees F. In a baking dish, combine first 6 ingredients and 1/2 of the sea salt.
- ❖ Cover with aluminum foil. Bake 20 minutes in the oven. Combine the asparagus, oil and salt.

- ❖ Cover and bake for about 15 minutes, or until the root vegetables become tender. Increase oven temperature to 450 degrees F.
- ❖ Remove aluminum foil and bake for 8 minutes, until potatoes are lightly browned.

26) BAKED KOHLRABI, YUCCA ROOT AND MUSTARD

Preparation Time:	Cooking Time:	Servings:

Ingredients:

- ✓ 1/2 pound kohlrabi, chopped
- ✓ ½ pound yucca root, chopped
- ✓ ½ pound mustard
- ✓ 2 tablespoons extra-virgin olive oil
- ✓ 12 garlic cloves, thinly sliced

Ingredients:

- ✓ 1 tablespoon and 1 teaspoon dried rosemary
- ✓ 4 teaspoons dried thyme
- ✓ 2 teaspoons sea salt
- ✓ 1 bunch fresh green beans, trimmed and cut into 1-inch pieces

- ❖ Preheat oven to 425 degrees F. In a baking dish, combine first 7 ingredients and 1/2 of the sea salt.
- ❖ Cover with aluminum foil. Bake 20 minutes in the oven. Combine the green beans, olive oil and salt.

- ❖ Cover and bake for about 15 minutes, or until root vegetables become tender. Increase the oven temperature to 450 degrees F.
- ❖ Remove the aluminum foil and bake for 8 minutes, until the potatoes become lightly browned.

27) BAKED PURPLE CABBAGE WITH RAINBOW PEPPERCORNS

Preparation Time:	Cooking Time:	Servings:

Ingredients:

- ✓ 1 (16-ounce) package of fresh purple cabbage
- ✓ 2 small red onions, thinly sliced
- ✓ 1/2 cup and 1 tablespoon extra virgin olive oil, divided
- ✓ 1/4 teaspoon sea salt

Ingredients:

- ✓ 1/4 teaspoon rainbow pepper
- ✓ 1 shallot, chopped
- ✓ 1/4 cup balsamic vinegar
- ✓ 1 teaspoon Herbes de Provence

Directions:

- ❖ Preheat oven to 425 degrees F (220 degrees C).
- ❖ Grease a baking dish. Combine the cabbage and onion in a bowl
- ❖ Add 4 tablespoons olive oil, salt and peppercorns Stir to coat and spread the sprout mixture on the baking sheet.

- ❖ Bake until sprouts and onion are tender, about 25-30 minutes. Heat the remaining tablespoon of olive oil in a small skillet over medium-high heat Sauté the shallots until tender, about 5 minutes.
- ❖ Add the balsamic vinegar and cook until the glaze is reduced, about 5 minutes.
- ❖ Add the Herbes de Provence into the balsamic glaze and pour over the sprouts.

28) BAKED CRIMINI MUSHROOMS AND RED POTATOES

Preparation Time:	Cooking Time:	Servings:

Ingredients:

- ✓ 1 pound red potatoes, cut in half
- ✓ 2 tablespoons extra virgin olive oil
- ✓ 1/2 pound cremini mushrooms
- ✓ 8 cloves unpeeled garlic
- ✓ 2 tablespoons chopped fresh thyme

Ingredients:

- ✓ 1 tablespoon extra virgin olive oil sea salt and ground black pepper to taste
- ✓ 1/4 pound cherry tomatoes
- ✓ 3 tablespoons toasted pine nuts
- ✓ 1/4 pound spinach, thinly sliced

Directions:

- ❖ Preheat oven to 425 degrees F. Spread potatoes in a skillet with 2 tablespoons olive oil and roast for 15 minutes, turning once.
- ❖ Add mushrooms with stem side up Add garlic cloves to skillet and cook until lightly browned Sprinkle with thyme.

- ❖ Drizzle with 1 tablespoon olive oil and season with sea salt and black pepper.
- ❖ Return to oven and bake for 5 minutes. Add the cherry tomatoes to the pan. Return to oven and bake until mushrooms are softened, 5 minutes.
- ❖ Sprinkle the pine nuts over the potatoes and mushrooms. Serve with the spinach.

29) CHAMPIGNON MUSHROOMS AND BAKED SUMMER SQUASH

Preparation Time:	Cooking Time:	Servings:

Ingredients:

- ✓ 1 pound summer squash, halved
- ✓ 2 tablespoons extra virgin olive oil
- ✓ 1/2 pound button mushrooms
- ✓ 8 cloves unpeeled garlic
- ✓ 2 tablespoons cumin
- ✓ 1 tablespoon annatto seeds

Ingredients:

- ✓ ½ tablespoon cayenne pepper
- ✓ 1 tablespoon extra virgin olive oil sea salt and ground black pepper to taste
- ✓ 1/4 pound cherry tomatoes
- ✓ 3 tablespoons toasted pine nuts
- ✓ 1/4 pound thinly sliced spinach

Directions:

- ❖ Preheat oven to 425 degrees F. Spread summer squash in a skillet with 2 tablespoons olive oil and roast for 15 minutes, turning once.
- ❖ Add mushrooms stem side up Add garlic cloves to skillet and cook until lightly browned Sprinkle with cumin, cayenne pepper and annatto seeds.

- ❖ Drizzle with 1 tablespoon olive oil and season with sea salt and black pepper.
- ❖ Return to oven and bake for 5 minutes. Add the cherry tomatoes to the skillet.
- ❖ Return to oven and bake until mushrooms are softened, 5 minutes.
- ❖ Sprinkle pine nuts over the summer squash and mushrooms. Serve with the spinach.

30) ROASTED WATERCRESS AND SUMMER SQUASH

Preparation Time:	Cooking Time:	Servings:

Ingredients:

- ✓ 1 1/2 pounds summer squash, peeled and cut into 1-inch chunks
- ✓ ½ red onion, thinly sliced
- ✓ ¼ cup water
- ✓ ½ vegetable stock cube, crumbled
- ✓ 1 tablespoon sesame oil

Ingredients:

- ✓ ½ teaspoon Chinese 5-spice powder
- ✓ ½ teaspoon Sichuan pepper
- ✓ ½ teaspoon chili powder Black pepper
- ✓ ½ pound fresh watercress, coarsely chopped

Directions:

- ❖ Place all ingredients in a saucepan over low heat except for the last one.
- ❖ Add a handful of watercress and fill the pot on low heat. If you can't put everything in at once, let the first batch cook first and add more watercress.

- ❖ Cook for 3 to 4 hours over medium heat until the summer squash is soft. Scrape down the sides and serve.

31) BUTTERED POTATOES AND SPINACH

Preparation Time:	Cooking Time:	Servings:

Ingredients:

- ✓ 1 1/2 pounds red potatoes, peeled and cut into 1-inch pieces
- ✓ ½ onion, thinly sliced
- ✓ ¼ cup water
- ✓ ½ vegetable stock cube, crumbled
- ✓ 2 tablespoons salted butter

Ingredients:

- ✓ ½ teaspoon Herbes de Provence
- ✓ ½ teaspoon thyme
- ✓ ½ teaspoon chili powder Black pepper
- ✓ ½ pound fresh spinach, coarsely chopped

❖ Place all ingredients in a pot over low heat except for the last one.
❖ Top with handfuls of spinach and fill the pot over low heat. If you can't put everything in at once, let the first batch cook first and add more spinach.

❖ Cook for 3 to 4 hours over medium heat until potatoes are soft. Scrape down the sides and serve.

32) SMOKED ROASTED BEETS AND CAULIFLOWER

Preparation Time:	Cooking Time:	Servings:

Ingredients:

- ✓ 1 1/2 pounds cauliflower, peeled and cut into 1-inch chunks ½ red onion, thinly sliced
- ✓ ¼ cup water
- ✓ ½ vegetable stock cube, crumbled
- ✓ 1 tablespoon extra-virgin olive oil

Ingredients:

- ✓ ½ teaspoon cumin
- ✓ ½ teaspoon chili powder Black pepper
- ✓ ½ pound fresh beets, coarsely chopped

❖ Place all ingredients in a saucepan over low heat except for the last one.
❖ Add a handful of chard and fill the pot over low heat. If you can't put everything in at once, let the first batch cook first and add more chard.

❖ Cook for 3 to 4 hours over medium heat until potatoes are soft.
❖ Scrape down the sides and serve.

33) ROASTED SPINACH AND BROCCOLI WITH JALAPENO

Preparation Time:	Cooking Time:	Servings:

Ingredients:

- ✓ 1 1/2 pounds broccoli florets
- ✓ ½ onion, thinly sliced
- ✓ ¼ cup water
- ✓ ½ vegetable stock cube, crumbled
- ✓ 1 tablespoon extra-virgin olive oil

Ingredients:

- ✓ ½ teaspoon cumin
- ✓ 8 jalapeno peppers, finely chopped
- ✓ 1 ancho chili pepper
- ✓ ½ teaspoon hot pepper powder Black pepper
- ✓ ½ pound fresh spinach, coarsely chopped

❖ Place all ingredients in a pot over low heat except for the last one.
❖ Top with handfuls of spinach and fill the pot over low heat. If you can't put everything in at once, let the first batch cook first and add more spinach.

❖ Cook for 3 to 4 hours over medium heat until broccoli is soft.
❖ Scrape down the sides and serve.

34) OMELETTE WITH ONIONS AND MUSHROOMS

Preparation Time: 15 minutes	**Cooking Time**:	**Servings**: 2

Ingredients:

- ✓ 4 eggs, beaten
- ✓ 1 cup mushrooms, sliced
- ✓ 2 tablespoons olive oil, divided

Ingredients:

- ✓ 1 clove garlic, minced Salt and black pepper to taste
- ✓ ¼ cup sliced onions

Directions:

- ❖ Heat the olive oil in a skillet over medium heat.
- ❖ Add the garlic, mushrooms and onions.
- ❖ Cook for 6 minutes, stirring often. Season with salt and pepper. Increase heat and cook for 3 minutes.

- ❖ Remove to a plate. In the same skillet, add the eggs and make sure they are evenly distributed.
- ❖ Add the vegetables. Cut into slices and serve.

35) GREEN CITRUS JUICE

Preparation Time: 5 minutes	**Cooking Time**:	**Servings**: 1

Ingredients:

- ✓ ½ grapefruit
- ✓ ½ lemon
- ✓ 3 cups kale
- ✓ 1 cucumber

Ingredients:

- ✓ ¼ cup fresh parsley leaves
- ✓ ¼ cup pineapple, cut into wedges
- ✓ ½ green apple
- ✓ 1 teaspoon fresh grated ginger

Directions:

- ❖ In a blender, place the kale, parsley, cucumber, pineapple, grapefruit, apple, lemon and ginger and blend until smooth.

- ❖ Serve in a tall glass.

36) ZUCCHINI AND EGG NESTS WITH CHILLI PEPPERS

Preparation Time: 25 minutes	**Cooking Time**:	**Servings**: 4

Ingredients:

- ✓ 4 eggs
- ✓ 2 tablespoons olive oil
- ✓ 1 pound zucchini, shredded Salt and black pepper to taste

Ingredients:

- ✓ ½ red pepper, seeded and chopped
- ✓ 2 tablespoons parsley, chopped

Directions:

- ❖ Preheat oven to 360 F. Combine the zucchini, salt, pepper and olive oil in a bowl.
- ❖ Form nests with a spoon on a greased baking sheet.

- ❖ Crack an egg into each nest and season with salt, pepper and chili. Bake for 11 minutes.
- ❖ Serve topped with parsley.

37) OATS WITH CHIA AND BANANA

Preparation Time: 10 minutes	Cooking Time:	Servings:

Ingredients:

- ✓ ½ cup walnuts, chopped
- ✓ 1 banana, peeled and sliced
- ✓ 1 cup Greek yogurt

Directions:

- ❖ Place the banana, yogurt, dates, cocoa powder, oats and chia seeds in a bowl and blend until smooth.
- ❖

Ingredients:

- ✓ 2 dates, pitted and chopped
- ✓ 1 cup rolled oats
- ✓ 2 tablespoons chia seeds

- ❖ Let stand for 1 hour and spoon onto a bowl.
- ❖ Sprinkle with walnuts and serve.

38) PARMESAN OMELETTE

Preparation Time: 5 minutes	Cooking Time: 10 minutes	Servings: 2

Ingredients:

- ✓ 1 tablespoon cream cheese
- ✓ 2 eggs, beaten
- ✓ ¼ teaspoon paprika
- ✓ ½ teaspoon dried oregano

Directions:

- ❖ Mix together the cream cheese with the eggs, dried oregano and dill.
- ❖ Place the coconut oil in a skillet and heat it until it coats the entire skillet.
- ❖ Then pour the egg mixture into the skillet and flatten it out.

Ingredients:

- ✓ ¼ teaspoon dried dill
- ✓ 1 oz Parmesan cheese, grated
- ✓ 1 teaspoon coconut oil

- ❖ Add the grated Parmesan cheese and close the lid. Cook the omelet for 10 minutes on low heat.
- ❖ Then transfer the cooked omelet to a serving plate and sprinkle with paprika.

39) WATERMELON PIZZA

Preparation Time: 10 minutes	Cooking Time:	Servings: 2

Ingredients:

- ✓ 9 ounces watermelon slice
- ✓ 1 tablespoon pomegranate sauce
- ✓

Directions:

- ❖ Place watermelon slice on plate and sprinkle with crumbled feta cheese.
- ❖ Add the fresh cilantro. After this, generously sprinkle the pizza with the pomegranate juice.
- ❖

Ingredients:

- ✓ 2 ounces feta cheese, crumbled
- ✓ 1 tablespoon fresh cilantro, chopped
- ✓

- ❖ Cut the pizza into portions.
- ❖

40) AVOCADO MILK SMOOTHIE

Preparation Time: 10 minutes	**Cooking Time**:	**Servings: 3**

Ingredients:

- ✓ 1 avocado, peeled, pitted
- ✓ 2 tablespoons liquid honey
- ✓ ½ teaspoon vanilla extract

Ingredients:

- ✓ ½ cup heavy cream
- ✓ 1 cup milk
- ✓ 1/3 cup ice cubes

Directions:

- ❖ Chop avocado and place in food processor.
- ❖ Add the liquid honey, vanilla extract, heavy cream, milk and ice cubes. Blend the mixture until smooth.

- ❖ Pour the cooked smoothie into serving glasses.

41) CAULIFLOWER FRITTERS

Preparation Time: 10 minutes	**Cooking Time**: 10 minutes	**Servings: 2**

Ingredients:

- ✓ 1 cup cauliflower, shredded
- ✓ 1 egg, beaten
- ✓ 1 tablespoon wheat flour, whole wheat

Ingredients:

- ✓ 1 oz parmesan cheese, grated
- ✓ ½ teaspoon ground black pepper
- ✓ 1 tablespoon canola oil

Directions:

- ❖ In the mixing bowl, stir together the shredded cauliflower and egg. Add the wheat flour, grated Parmesan cheese and ground black pepper.
- ❖ Mix the mixture with the help of a fork until it is smooth and homogeneous.

- ❖ Pour the canola oil into the pan and bring it to a boil. Cut out pancakes from the cauliflower mixture with the help of fingertips or a spoon and transfer them to the hot oil.
- ❖ Roast the fritters for 4 minutes on each side over medium-low heat.

42) COCOA OATMEAL

Preparation Time: 10 minutes	**Cooking Time**: 15 minutes	**Servings: 2**

Ingredients:

- ✓ 1 ½ cups oatmeal
- ✓ 1 tablespoon cocoa powder
- ✓ ½ cup heavy cream
- ✓ ¼ cup water

Ingredients:

- ✓ 1 teaspoon vanilla extract
- ✓ 1 tablespoon butter
- ✓ 2 tablespoons Splenda

Directions:

- ❖ Mix together the oatmeal with the cocoa powder and Splenda.
- ❖ Transfer the mixture to the saucepan, add the vanilla extract, water and heavy cream.

- ❖ Stir gently with the help of the spatula. Close the lid and cook for 10-15 minutes over medium-low heat.
- ❖ Remove the cocoa baked oatmeal from the heat and add the butter. Stir well.

43) SPANAKOPITA BREAKFAST

Preparation Time: 15 minutes	**Cooking Time:** 1 hour	**Servings:** 6

Ingredients:

- ✓ 2 cups spinach
- ✓ 1 white onion, diced
- ✓ ½ cup fresh parsley
- ✓ 1 teaspoon minced garlic
- ✓ 3 ounces feta cheese, crumbled

Ingredients:

- ✓ 1 teaspoon paprika powder
- ✓ 2 eggs, beaten
- ✓ 1/3 cup butter, melted
- ✓ 2 ounces Phyllo dough

Directions:

- ❖ Separate the Phyllo dough into 2 parts.
- ❖ Brush the casserole mold well with butter and place 1 part Phyllo dough inside.
- ❖ Brush its surface with butter as well. Place the spinach and fresh parsley in the blender.

- ❖ Blend until smooth and transfer to the bowl. Add the minced garlic, feta cheese, ground paprika, eggs and diced onion.
- ❖ Mix well. Spoon the spinach mixture into the casserole dish and flatten well.
- ❖ Cover the spinach mixture with the remaining Phyllo dough and pour the remaining butter over it.
- ❖ Bake the spanakopita for 1 hour at 350F. Cut into portions.

44) FRITATTA OF POBLANO

Preparation Time: 10 minutes	**Cooking Time:** 15 minutes	**Servings:** 4

Ingredients:

- ✓ 5 eggs, beaten
- ✓ 1 poblano pepper, chopped, raw
- ✓ 1 oz shallots, chopped
- ✓ 1/3 cup heavy cream

Ingredients:

- ✓ ½ teaspoon butter
- ✓ ½ teaspoon salt
- ✓ ½ teaspoon chili flakes
- ✓ 1 tablespoon fresh cilantro, chopped

Directions:

- ❖ Mix together the eggs with the heavy cream and beat until smooth.
- ❖ Add the chopped chile poblano, scallions, salt, chili flakes and fresh cilantro.

- ❖ Place the butter in a skillet and melt it. Add the egg mixture and flatten it in the pan if necessary.
- ❖ Close the lid and cook the omelet for 15 minutes over medium-low heat. When the omelet is cooked, it will be firm.

45) SIMPLE AND FAST STEAK

Preparation Time: 15 minutes	**Cooking Time:** 10 minutes	**Servings:** 2

Ingredients:

- ✓ • ½ pound of steak, quality cut

Ingredients:

- ✓ Salt and freshly cracked black pepper

Directions:

- ❖ Turn on the air fryer, put on the frying basket, then set the temperature to 385°F and let it preheat.
- ❖ Meanwhile, prepare the steaks, and for that, season them with salt and freshly cracked black pepper on both sides.
- ❖ When the fryer is preheated, add the prepared steaks into the fryer basket, close it with the lid and cook for 15 minutes.

- ❖ When done, transfer the steaks to a plate and serve immediately. To prepare the meal, divide the steaks evenly between two heat-resistant containers, close them with the lid and refrigerate for up to 3 days until ready to serve.
- ❖ When ready to eat, reheat the steaks in the microwave until hot and then serve.

46) ZUCCHINI TAGLIATELLE WITH FOUR CHEESES AND BASIL PESTO

Preparation Time: 10 minutes	**Cooking Time**: 15 minutes	**Servings: 2**

Ingredients:

- ✓ 4 cups zucchini noodles
- ✓ 4 ounces mascarpone cheese
- ✓ 1/8 cup Romano cheese
- ✓ 2 tablespoons grated Parmesan cheese
- ✓ ¼ teaspoon salt

Ingredients:

- ✓ ½ teaspoon ground black pepper
- ✓ 2 1/8 teaspoon nutmeg powder
- ✓ 1/8 cup basil pesto
- ✓ ½ cup shredded mozzarella cheese
- ✓ 1 tablespoon olive oil

Directions:

- ❖ Turn on the oven, then set the temperature to 400°F and let it preheat.
- ❖ Meanwhile, place the zucchini noodles in a heat-resistant bowl and microwave on high heat for 3 minutes, set aside until needed. Take another heat-resistant bowl, add all the cheeses except the mozzarella, season with salt, black pepper and nutmeg, and microwave on high heat for 1 minute until the cheese has melted.

- ❖ Blend the cheese mixture, add the cooked zucchini noodles along with the basil pesto and mozzarella and fold until well mixed.
- ❖ Take a casserole dish, grease it with oil, add the zucchini noodle mixture and then bake for 10 minutes. Serve immediately.

47) BLUEBERRY AND VANILLA SCONES

Preparation Time: 10 minutes	**Cooking Time**: 10 minutes	**Servings: 12**

Ingredients:

- ✓ 1½ cups almond flour
- ✓ 3 organic eggs, beaten
- ✓ 2 tablespoons baking powder
- ✓ ½ cup stevia

Ingredients:

- ✓ 2 tablespoons vanilla extract, unsweetened
- ✓ ¾ cup fresh raspberries
- ✓ 1 tablespoon olive oil

Directions:

- ❖ Turn on the oven, then set the temperature to 375°F and let it preheat.
- ❖ Take a large bowl, add the flour and eggs, stir in the baking powder, stevia and vanilla until combined and then add the berries.

- ❖ Take a baking sheet, grease it with oil, pour the prepared batter on top with an ice cream scoop and bake for 10 minutes until cooked through.
- ❖ When done, transfer the scones to a wire rack, let them cool completely and then serve.

48) FANTASTIC COFFEE WITH BUTTER

Preparation Time: 5 minutes	**Cooking Time**: 5 minutes	**Servings: 1**

Ingredients:

- ✓ 1 cup water
- ✓ 1 tablespoon coconut oil

Ingredients:

- ✓ 1 tablespoon unsalted butter
- ✓ 2 tablespoons coffee

Directions:

- ❖ Take a small skillet, place it on medium heat, pour in the water and bring to a boil.
- ❖ Then add the remaining ingredients, stir well and cook until the butter and oil have melted.

- ❖ Remove the pan from the heat, strain the coffee through a strainer and serve immediately.

49) SCRAMBLED EGGS

Preparation Time: 25 minutes	Cooking Time:	Servings: 2

Ingredients:	Ingredients:
✓ 1 tablespoon butter	✓ 4 eggs Salt and black pepper, to taste

Directions:

❖ Combine eggs, salt and black pepper together in a bowl and set aside.

❖ Heat the butter in a skillet over medium-low heat and slowly add the beaten eggs.

❖ Stir the eggs in the pan continuously with the help of a fork for about 4 minutes. Distribute onto a plate and serve immediately.

50) CREAMY PARSLEY SOUFFLÉ

Preparation Time: 25 minutes	Cooking Time:	Servings: 2

Ingredients:	Ingredients:
✓ 2 fresh red peppers, chopped Salt, to taste ✓ 4 eggs	✓ 4 tablespoons light cream ✓ 2 tablespoons fresh parsley, chopped

Directions:

❖ Preheat oven to 375 degrees F and grease 2 souffle dishes.

❖ Combine all ingredients in a bowl and mix well. Spoon the mixture into the prepared souffle dishes and transfer to the oven.

❖ Bake for about 6 minutes and serve immediately.

❖ To prepare the meal, you can refrigerate this creamy parsley soufflé in the ramekins covered with aluminum foil for about 2-3 days.

51) CINNAMON FAUX-ST CRUNCH CEREAL

Preparation Time: 35 minutes	Cooking Time:	Servings: 2

Ingredients:	Ingredients:
✓ ¼ cup hulled hemp seeds ✓ ½ tablespoon coconut oil ✓ ¼ cup ground flax seeds	✓ 1 tablespoon ground cinnamon ✓ ¼ cup apple juice

Directions:

❖ Preheat oven to 300 degrees F and line a cookie sheet with baking paper.

❖ Place the hemp seeds, flax seeds and ground cinnamon in a food processor.

❖ Add the coconut oil and apple juice and blend until smooth. Pour the mixture onto the cookie sheet and transfer to the oven.

❖ Bake for about 15 minutes and lower the oven temperature to 250 degrees F.

❖ Bake for another 10 minutes and turn the dish out of the oven, turning it off.

❖ Cut into small squares and place in the oven turned off. Place the cereal in the oven for 1 hour until crispy. Unmold and serve with unsweetened almond milk.

52) OATMEAL AND CARROT CUPCAKES

Total Time: 30 minutes	Cooking Time:	Servings: 6

Ingredients:

- ✓ 1 ½ cups grated carrots
- ✓ ¼ cup pecans, chopped
- ✓ 1 cup oat bran
- ✓ 1 cup whole-wheat flour
- ✓ ½ cup all-purpose flour
- ✓ ½ cup old-fashioned oats
- ✓ 3 tablespoons light brown sugar
- ✓ 1 tablespoon vanilla extract
- ✓ ½ lemon, peeled

Ingredients:

- ✓ 1 tablespoon baking powder
- ✓ 2 tablespoons cinnamon powder
- ✓ 2 tablespoons ginger powder
- ✓ ½ tablespoon nutmeg powder
- ✓ ¼ salt
- ✓ 1¼ cup soy milk
- ✓ 2 tablespoons honey
- ✓ 1 egg
- ✓ 2 tablespoons olive oil

Directions:

- ❖ Preheat oven to 350 F and grease two paper-lined muffin pans with cooking spray.
- ❖ Mix whole wheat flour, all-purpose flour, oat bran, oats, sugar, baking powder, cinnamon, nutmeg, ginger and salt in a bowl; set aside.
- ❖ Beat egg with soy milk, honey, vanilla, lemon zest and olive oil in another bowl.

- ❖ Pour this mixture into the flour mixture and combine to blend, leaving some lumps.
- ❖ Stir in carrots and pecans. Spoon batter into each muffin cup lined 3/4 way up. Bake for about 20 minutes.
- ❖ Poke with a toothpick and if it comes out easily, the cakes are cooked. Allow to cool and serve.

53) STRAWBERRY AND CHOCOLATE SMOOTHIE

Preparation Time: 5 minutes	Cooking Time:	Servings: 2

Ingredients:

- ✓ 1 cup buttermilk
- ✓ 2 cups strawberries, hulled
- ✓ 1 cup crushed ice
- ✓

Ingredients:

- ✓ 3 tablespoons cocoa powder
- ✓ 3 tablespoons honey
- ✓ 2 mint leaves
- ✓

Directions:

- ❖ In a food processor, juice the buttermilk, strawberries, ice, cocoa powder, mint and honey until smooth. Serve.
- ❖

54) CAULIFLOWER OMELETTE WITH CHEESE

Preparation Time: 30 minutes	**Cooking Time**:	**Servings**: 4

Ingredients:

- ✓ 2 tablespoons olive oil
- ✓ ½ pound cauliflower florets
- ✓ ½ cup skim milk
- ✓ 6 eggs
- ✓

Ingredients:

- ✓ 1 red bell pepper, seeded and chopped
- ✓ ½ cup fontina cheese, grated
- ✓ ½ teaspoon red pepper
- ✓ ½ teaspoon turmeric Salt and black pepper to taste
- ✓

Directions:

- ❖ Preheat oven to 360 F. In a bowl, beat the eggs with the milk.
- ❖ Add the fontina cheese, red pepper, turmeric, salt and pepper. Stir in the red bell pepper.
- ❖ Heat the olive oil in a skillet over medium heat and pour in the egg mixture; cook for 4-5 minutes. Set aside.

- ❖ Blanch cauliflower florets in a saucepan for 5 minutes until tender. Spread over egg mixture.
- ❖ Place the pan in the oven and bake for 15 minutes or until set and golden brown. Allow to cool for a few minutes before slicing. Serve in slices.

55) MOZZARELLA AND OLIVES CILANTRO CAKES

Preparation Time: 25 minutes	**Cooking Time**:	**Servings**: 6

Ingredients:

- ✓ ¼ cup mozzarella, shredded
- ✓ ¼ cup black olives, pitted and chopped
- ✓ ½ cup low-fat milk
- ✓ 4 tablespoons coconut oil, softened
- ✓ 1 egg, beaten
- ✓ 1 cup cornmeal

Ingredients:

- ✓ 1 teaspoon baking powder
- ✓ 3 sun-dried tomatoes, finely chopped
- ✓ 2 tablespoons fresh parsley, chopped
- ✓ 2 tablespoons fresh cilantro, chopped
- ✓ ¼ teaspoon kosher salt

Directions:

- ❖ Preheat oven to 360 F. In a bowl, beat the egg with the milk and coconut oil. In a separate bowl, mix the salt, cornmeal, cilantro and baking powder.

- ❖ Combine the wet ingredients with the dry mixture. Stir in the black olives, tomatoes, herbs and mozzarella cheese.
- ❖ Pour the mixture into greased ramekins and bake for about 18-20 minutes or until cooked and golden brown.

56) MUSHROOM AND QUINOA CUPS		
Preparation Time: 40 minutes	**Cooking Time**:	**Servings**: 6

Ingredients:

- ✓ 6 eggs
- ✓ 1 cup quinoa, cooked Salt and black pepper to taste
- ✓ 1 cup Gruyere cheese, grated
- ✓

Ingredients:

- ✓ 1 small yellow onion, chopped
- ✓ 1 cup mushrooms, sliced
- ✓ ½ cup green olives, chopped
- ✓

Directions:

- ❖ Whisk eggs, salt, pepper, Gruyere cheese, onion, mushrooms and green olives in a bowl.
- ❖

- ❖ Pour into a silicone muffin pan and bake for 30 minutes at 360 F. Serve warm.

57) CLASSIC SPANISH TORTILLA		
Preparation Time: 35 minutes	**Cooking Time**:	**Servings**: 4

Ingredients:

- ✓ 1 ½ lb. golden potatoes, peeled and sliced
- ✓ 1 sweet onion, thinly sliced
- ✓ 8 eggs

Ingredients:

- ✓ ½ dried oregano
- ✓ ½ cup olive oil Salt to taste

Directions:

- ❖ Heat olive oil in a skillet over medium heat. Fry the potatoes for 8-10 minutes, stirring often.
- ❖ Add the onion and salt and cook for 5-6 minutes until the potatoes are tender and lightly browned; set aside. In a bowl, beat eggs with a pinch of salt.

- ❖ Add the potato mixture and mix well. Pour into the skillet and cook for about 10-12 minutes. Flip the tortilla with a plate and cook for another 2 minutes until nice and crispy.
- ❖ Cut into slices and serve warm.

58) EGG CAKES WITH ZUCCHINI AND MUSHROOMS

Preparation Time: 20 minutes	Cooking Time:	Servings: 4

Ingredients:

- ✓ 1 cup Parmesan cheese, grated
- ✓ 1 onion, chopped
- ✓ 1 cup mushrooms, sliced
- ✓ 1 red bell pepper, chopped

Ingredients:

- ✓ 1 zucchini, chopped Salt and black pepper to taste
- ✓ 8 eggs, beaten
- ✓ 1 tablespoon olive oil
- ✓ 2 tablespoons chives, chopped

Directions:

- ❖ 1 zucchini, chopped Salt and black pepper to taste
- ❖ 8 eggs, beaten
- ❖ 1 tablespoon olive oil
- ❖ 2 tablespoons chives, chopped
- ❖ Preheat the oven to 360 F. Heat the olive oil in a skillet over medium heat and sauté the onion, zucchini, mushrooms, salt and pepper for 5 minutes until tender.

- ❖ Spread the mixture into the muffin cups and add the eggs. Sprinkle with salt, pepper and chives and bake for 10 minutes.
- ❖ Serve immediately.

59) SCRAMBLED EGG WITH ANCHOVIES

Preparation Time: 20 minutes	Cooking Time:	Servings: 4

Ingredients:

- ✓ 2 tablespoons olive oil
- ✓ 1 chopped green bell pepper
- ✓ 2 chopped anchovy fillets
- ✓ 8 diced cherry tomatoes
- ✓ 2 chopped spring onions

Ingredients:

- ✓ 1 tablespoon drained capers
- ✓ 5 pitted and sliced black olives
- ✓ 6 beaten eggs Salt and black pepper to taste
- ✓ ¼ teaspoon dried oregano
- ✓ 1 tablespoon chopped parsley

Directions:

- ❖ Heat the olive oil in a skillet over medium heat and cook the bell bell pepper and spring onions for 3 minutes.

- ❖ Add the anchovies, cherry tomatoes, capers and black olives and cook for another 2 minutes.
- ❖ Add the eggs and sprinkle with salt, pepper and oregano and scramble for 5 minutes. Serve sprinkled with parsley.

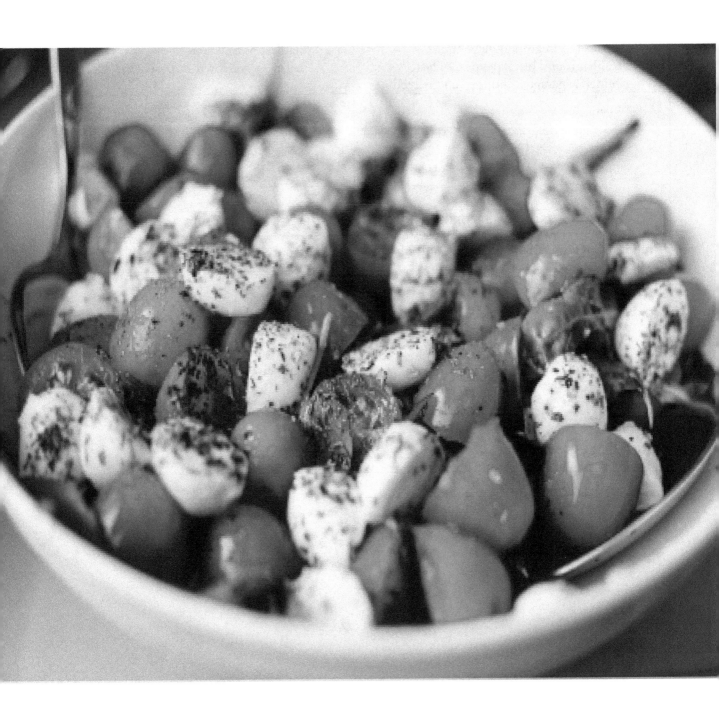

63) BEEF WITH ASPARAGUS AND PEPPERS

Preparation Time: 15 minutes	Cooking Time: 13 minutes	Servings: 4-5

Ingredients:

- ✓ 4 cloves garlic, minced
- ✓ - 3 tablespoons coconut aminos
- ✓ - 1/8 teaspoon red pepper flakes, crushed
- ✓ - 1/8 teaspoon ground ginger
- ✓ - Freshly ground black pepper, to taste
- ✓ - 1 bunch asparagus, chopped and halved

Ingredients:

- ✓ - 2 tablespoons olive oil, divided
- ✓ - 1 pound steak, cut and thinly sliced
- ✓ - 1 red bell pepper, seeded and sliced
- ✓ - 3 tablespoons water
- ✓ - 2 teaspoons arrowroot powder

Directions:

❖ In a bowl, mix together garlic, coconut aminos, red pepper flakes, crushed and ground ginger, and black pepper. Keep aside. In a pot of boiling water, cook asparagus for about 2 minutes. Drain and rinse under cold water. In a substantial skillet, heat 1 tablespoon oil over medium-high heat.

❖ Add the beef and sauté for about 3-4 minutes. Using a slotted spoon, transfer the beef to a bowl. In a similar skillet, heat the remaining oil over medium heat. Add the asparagus and bell bell pepper and sauté for about 2-3 minutes.

❖ Meanwhile in the bowl, mix together the water and arrowroot powder. Stir in the beef, garlic mixture and arrowroot mixture and cook for about 3-4 minutes or until desired thickness.

64) GROUND BEEF WITH CASHEWS AND VEGETABLES

Preparation Time: 15 minutes	Cooking Time: quarter hour	Servings: 4

Ingredients:

- ✓ 1½ pounds lean ground beef
- ✓ - 1 tablespoon garlic, minced
- ✓ - 2 tablespoons fresh ginger, minced
- ✓ - ¼ cup coconut aminos
- ✓ - Salt and freshly ground black pepper, to taste

Ingredients:

- ✓ - 1 medium onion, sliced
- ✓ - 1 can water chestnuts, drained and sliced
- ✓ - 1 large green bell pepper, seeded and sliced
- ✓ - ½ cup raw cashews, toasted

Directions:

❖ Heat a nonstick skillet over medium-high heat. Add the beef and cook for about 6-8 minutes, breaking into pieces with the whole spoon.

❖ Add the garlic, ginger, coconut aminos, salt and black pepper and cook about 2 minutes. Add the vegetables and cook about 5 minutes or until desired doneness.

❖ Add cashews and immediately remove from heat. 6. Serve hot.

65) SPICY AND CREAMY GROUND BEEF CURRY		
Preparation Time: quarter hour	**Cooking Time**: 32 minutes	**Servings**: 4

Ingredients:

- ✓ 1-2 tablespoons coconut oil
- ✓ - 1 teaspoon black mustard seeds
- ✓ - 2 sprigs curry leaves
- ✓ - 1 Serrano bell pepper, chopped
- ✓ - 1 large red onion, finely chopped
- ✓ - 1 (1-inch) piece fresh ginger, chopped
- ✓ - 4 cloves garlic, chopped
- ✓ - 1 teaspoon ground coriander –
- ✓ 1 teaspoon ground cumin
- ✓ - ½ teaspoon ground turmeric

Ingredients:

- ✓ - ¼ teaspoon red chili powder
- ✓ - Salt, to taste
- ✓ - 1 pound lean ground beef
- ✓ - 1 potato, peeled and chopped
- ✓ - 3 medium carrots, peeled and chopped
- ✓ - ¼ cup water
- ✓ - 1 can coconut milk (14 ounces)
- ✓ - Salt and freshly ground black pepper, to taste
- ✓ - Fresh chopped cilantro, for garnish

Directions:

❖ In a large skillet, melt the coconut oil over medium heat. Add the mustard seeds and sauté for about thirty seconds. Add the curry leaves and Serrano pepper and sauté about half a minute. Add the onion, ginger and garlic and sauté for about 4-5 minutes.

❖ Add the spices and cook for about 1 minute. Add the beef and cook for about 4-5 minutes. Add the potato, carrot and water and simmer. Simmer, covered, for about 5 minutes. Add coconut milk and simmer for about fifteen minutes.

❖ Add salt and black pepper and remove from heat. Serve hot while using the cilantro garnish.

66) GRILLED BEEF STEAK IN PAN		
Preparation Time: 10 minutes	**Cooking Time**: 12-16 minutes	**Servings**: 3-4

Ingredients:

- ✓ 8 medium garlic cloves, crushed
- ✓ - 1 (5-inch) piece of fresh ginger, thinly sliced
- ✓ - 1 tablespoon organic honey

Ingredients:

- ✓ - ¼ cup organic olive oil
- ✓ - Salt and freshly ground black pepper, to taste
- ✓ - 1½ pounds of steak, chopped

Directions:

❖ In a large sealable bag, mix all ingredients except the steak. Add the steak and coat generously with the marinade. Seal the bag and refrigerate to marinate for about a day. Remove from refrigerator and at room temperature for about 15 minutes.

❖ Lightly grease a grill pan and heat over medium-high heat. Remove excess marinade from steak and place in grill pan. Cook for about 6-8 minutes on each side.

❖ Remove from grill pan and hold the side for about 10 minutes before slicing. Using a clear, crisp knife, cut into desired slices and serve.

67) LAMB WITH ZUCCHINI AND COUSCOUS

Preparation Time: 15 minutes	**Cooking Time**: 8 minutes	**Servings**: 2

Ingredients:

- ✓ ¾ cup couscous
- ✓ - ¾ cup boiling water
- ✓ - ¼ cup fresh cilantro, chopped
- ✓ - 1 tablespoon olive oil
- ✓ - 5 ounces lamb leg steak, cut into ¾-inch cubes
- ✓ - 1 medium zucchini, thinly sliced
- ✓ - 1 medium red onion, cut into wedges

Ingredients:

- ✓ - 1 teaspoon ground cumin
- ✓ - 1 teaspoon ground cilantro
- ✓ - ¼ teaspoon red pepper flakes, crushed
- ✓ - Salt, to taste
- ✓ - ¼ cup plain Greek yogurt
- ✓ - 1 garlic, minced

Directions:

- ❖ In a bowl, add couscous and boiling water and stir to combine. Cover while setting aside about 5 minutes. Add the cilantro and, using a fork, mash completely.

- ❖ Meanwhile, in a large skillet, heat oil over high heat. Add the lamb and sauté for about 2-3 minutes. Add the zucchini and onion and sauté for about 2 minutes.
- ❖ Add the spices and sauté for about 1 minute. Add the couscous and sauté for about 2 minutes. In a bowl, stir together the yogurt and garlic. Divide the lamb mixture evenly among the serving plates. Serve with the yogurt dressing.

68) ROAST LEG OF LAMB

Preparation Time: quarter hour	**Cooking Time**: 75-100 minutes	**Servings**: 8

Ingredients:

- ✓ 1/3 cup fresh parsley, chopped
- ✓ 4 cloves garlic, chopped
- ✓ 1 teaspoon fresh lemon zest, finely grated
- ✓ 1 tablespoon ground coriander
- ✓ 1 tablespoon ground cumin
- ✓ 1 teaspoon ground cinnamon

Ingredients:

- ✓ 1 teaspoon ground turmeric
- ✓ 1 tablespoon sweet paprika
- ✓ ½ teaspoon allspice
- ✓ 20 strands saffron, crushed
- ✓ 1/3 cup essential olive oil
- ✓ 1 5-pound leg of lamb, cut

Directions:

- ❖ In a bowl, mix all ingredients except the lamb. Generously coat the leg of lamb with the marinade mixture. Using plastic wrap, cover the leg of lamb and refrigerate to marinate for about 4-8 hours. Remove from refrigerator and hold at room temperature for about half an hour before roasting.

- ❖ Preheat the oven to 350 degrees F. Place the rack inside the center of the oven. Lightly, grease a roasting pan make a rack inside the pan. Place the lower limb of the lamb in the rack in the prepared roasting pan.
- ❖ Roast for about 75-100 minutes or until desired doneness, rotating once inside the middle.

69) GRILLED LAMB CHOPS

Preparation Time: 10 minutes	**Cooking Time:** 6 minutes	**Servings: 4**

Ingredients:

- ✓ 1 tablespoon fresh ginger, grated
- ✓ 4 cloves garlic, coarsely chopped
- ✓ 1 teaspoon ground cumin
- ✓ ½ teaspoon red chili powder

Ingredients:

- ✓ Salt and freshly ground black pepper, to taste
- ✓ 1 tablespoon essential olive oil
- ✓ 1 tablespoon fresh lemon juice
- ✓ 8 lamb chops, sliced

Directions:

- ❖ In a bowl, mix all ingredients except chops. Using a hand blender, blend until smooth. Add chops and coat generously with mixture. Refrigerate to marinate overnight.

- ❖ Preheat barbecue grill until hot. Grease the grill grate. Grill the chops for about 3 minutes per side.

70) FRESH LIME JUICE

Preparation Time: 15 minutes	**Cooking Time:** 13 minutes	**Servings: 4**

Ingredients:

- ✓ 1 tablespoon fresh ginger, finely chopped
- ✓ - 4 cloves garlic, finely chopped
- ✓ - 1 cup fresh cilantro, chopped and divided
- ✓ - ¼ cup plus 1 tablespoon olive oil, divided

Ingredients:

- ✓ - 1 pound 10-pound pork, chopped, thinly sliced
- ✓ - 2 onions, thinly sliced
- ✓ - 1 green bell pepper, seeded and thinly sliced
- ✓ - 1 tablespoon fresh lime juice

Directions:

- ❖ In a substantial bowl, stir together ginger, garlic, ½ cup cilantro and ¼ cup oil. - Add the pork and coat generously with the mixture. –
- ❖ Refrigerate to marinate for about a couple of hours. - Heat a large skillet over medium-high heat. - Add the pork mixture and sauté for about 4-5 minutes. - Transfer the pork to a bowl. - In the same skillet, heat the remaining oil over medium heat. –

- ❖ Add the onion and sauté for about 3 minutes. - Add bell bell pepper and sauté for about 3 minutes. - Stir in pork, lime juice and remaining cilantro and cook for about 2 minutes. - Serve hot.

71) GROUND PORK WITH WATER CHESTNUTS

Preparation Time: 15 minutes	**Cooking Time:** 12 minutes	**Servings: 4**

Ingredients:

- ✓ 1 tablespoon plus
- ✓ 1 teaspoon coconut oil
- ✓ - 1 tablespoon fresh ginger, chopped
- ✓ - 1 bunch shallots (white and green parts separated), chopped
- ✓ - 1 pound lean ground pork - Salt, to taste

Ingredients:

- ✓ - 1 tablespoon 5-spice powder
- ✓ - 1 can water chestnuts (18 ounces), drained and chopped
- ✓ - 1 tablespoon organic honey
- ✓ - 2 tablespoons fresh lime juice

- ❖ In a large, heavy-bottomed skillet, heat the oil over high heat. Add the ginger and scallion whites and sauté for about ½-1½ minutes. Add the pork and cook for about 4-5 minutes.

- ❖ Drain the extra fat from the pan. Add the salt and 5-spice powder and cook for about 2-3 minutes. Add the scallion greens and remaining ingredients and cook, stirring constantly for about 1-2 minutes.

72) CLEANED PARSLEY AND CHICKEN BREAST

Preparation Time: 10 minutes	**Cooking Time:** 40 minutes	**Servings: 2**

Ingredients:

- ✓ 1/2 tablespoon dried parsley
- ✓ 1/2 tablespoon dried basil
- ✓ 2 chicken breast halves, boneless and skinless

Ingredients:

- ✓ 1/4 teaspoon sunflower seeds
- ✓ 1/4 teaspoon red pepper flakes, crushed
- ✓ 1 tomato, sliced

Directions:

❖ Preheat the oven to 350 degrees F. Take a 9x13-inch baking dish and grease it with cooking spray. Sprinkle 1 tablespoon of parsley, 1 teaspoon of basil and spread the mixture on your baking sheet.

❖ Arrange the chicken breast halves on the baking sheet and sprinkle the garlic slices on top. Take a small bowl and add 1 teaspoon of parsley, 1 teaspoon of basil, sunflower seeds, basil, red pepper and mix well.

❖ Pour mixture over chicken breast. Top with tomato slices and cover, bake for 25 minutes. Remove cover and bake for an additional 15 minutes. Serve and enjoy!

73) HEARTY CHICKEN WITH LEMON AND PEPPER

Preparation Time: 5 minutes	**Cooking Time:** 15 minutes	**Servings: 4**

Ingredients:

- ✓ 2 teaspoons olive oil
- ✓ 1 ¼ pounds skinless chicken cutlets
- ✓ 2 whole eggs
- ✓ ¼ cup panko crumbs

Ingredients:

- ✓ 1 tablespoon lemon pepper Sunflower seeds and pepper to taste
- ✓ 3 cups green beans
- ✓ ¼ cup Parmesan cheese
- ✓ ¼ teaspoon garlic powder

Directions:

❖ Preheat oven to 425 degrees F. Take a bowl and stir in dressing, Parmesan cheese, lemon pepper, garlic powder, panko. Beat the eggs in another bowl.

❖ Coat cutlets in eggs and press into panko mixture. Transfer the coated chicken to a parchment lined baking sheet.

❖ Toss the beans in oil, pepper, add the sunflower seeds and arrange them on the side of the baking sheet. Bake for 15 minutes. Enjoy!

74) HEALTHY CARROT CHIPS

Preparation Time: 10 minutes	**Cooking Time:** 10 minutes	**Servings: 4**

Ingredients:

- ✓ 3 cups carrots, cut into thin rounds
- ✓ 2 tablespoons olive oil

Ingredients:

- ✓ 2 teaspoons ground cumin
- ✓ ½ teaspoon smoked paprika Pinch of sunflower seeds

Directions:

❖ Preheat oven to 400 degrees F. Slice carrot into paper-thin coins using a potato peeler. Place slices in a bowl and toss with oil and spices.

❖ Arrange slices on a baking sheet lined with parchment paper in a single layer. Sprinkle with sunflower seeds. Transfer to oven and bake for 8-10 minutes. Remove and serve. Enjoy!

75) AMAZING GRILLED CHICKEN AND BLUEBERRY SALAD

Preparation Time: 10 minutes	**Cooking Time**: 25 minutes	**Servings: 5**

Ingredients:	Ingredients:
For dressing ✓ ¼ cup olive oil ✓ ¼ cup apple cider vinegar ✓ ¼ cup blueberries ✓ 2 tablespoons honey Sunflower seeds and pepper to taste	✓ 5 cups mixed greens ✓ ù1 cup blueberries ✓ ¼ cup slivered almonds ✓ 2 cups chicken breasts, cooked and diced
Directions: ❖ take a bowl and add the veggies, berries, almonds, chicken cubes and mix well. Take a bowl and mix the dressing ingredients, pour the mix into a blender and blend until smooth.	❖ Add the dressing on top of the chicken cubes and mix well. Season more and enjoy!

76) ELEGANT PUMPKIN CHILI DISH

Preparation Time: 10 minutes	**Cooking Time**: 15 minutes	**Servings: 4**

Ingredients:	Ingredients:
✓ 3 cups yellow onion, minced ✓ 8 cloves garlic, minced ✓ 1 pound turkey, ground ✓ 2 cans (15 ounces each) roasted tomatoes ✓ 2 cups pumpkin puree	✓ 1 cup chicken broth ✓ 4 teaspoons chili spice ✓ 1 teaspoon cinnamon powder ✓ 1 teaspoon sea sunflower seeds
Directions: ❖ Take a large saucepan and place it over medium-high heat. Add the coconut oil and let the oil heat up. Add the onion and garlic, sauté for 5 minutes.	❖ Add ground turkey and break it up while cooking, cook for 5 minutes. Add remaining ingredients and bring mixture to a simmer. ❖ Simmer for 15 minutes (without a lid). Pour in the chicken broth. Serve with desired salad. Enjoy!

77) TASTY ROASTED BROCCOLI

Preparation Time: 5 minutes	**Cooking Time**: 20 minutes	**Servings: 4**

Ingredients:	Ingredients:
✓ 4 cups broccoli florets	✓ 1 tablespoon olive oil Sunflower seeds and pepper to taste
❖ Preheat oven to 400 degrees F. Add broccoli to a ziplock bag alongside the oil and shake until coated.	❖ Add the dressing and shake again. Spread broccoli on a baking sheet and bake for 20 minutes. Allow to cool and serve. Enjoy!

78) SOUTHWEST PORK CHOPS

Preparation Time: 10 minutes	**Cooking Time**: 15 minutes	**Servings: 4**

Ingredients:

- ✓ Cooking spray if needed
- ✓ 4-ounce pork chop, boneless and fat-free
- ✓ 1/3 cup sauce

Ingredients:

- ✓ 2 tablespoons fresh lime juice
- ✓ ¼ cup fresh cilantro, chopped

Directions:

- ❖ Take a large nonstick skillet and spray it with cooking spray. Heat until hot over high heat. Press the chops with the palm of your hand to flatten them slightly.

- ❖ Add them to the skillet and cook 1 minute on each side until golden brown. Lower the heat to medium-low. Combine the salsa and lime juice.

- ❖ Pour the mixture over the chops. Simmer uncovered for about 8 minutes until chops are perfectly cooked. Sprinkle a little cilantro on top if needed. Serve.

79) CHICKEN SAUCE

Preparation Time: 4 minutes	**Cooking Time**: 14 minutes	**Servings: 1**

Ingredients:

- ✓ 2 chicken breasts
- ✓ 1 cup salsa
- ✓ 1 taco seasoning mix

Ingredients:

- ✓ 1 cup plain Greek yogurt
- ✓ ½ cup annealed kite/cashew cheese, cubed

Directions:

- ❖ Take a skillet and place it over medium heat. Add the chicken breast, ½ cup of salsa and taco seasoning.

- ❖ Stir well and cook for 12-15 minutes until chicken is done. Remove chicken and cut into cubes. Place cubes on a toothpick and top with cheddar. Place yogurt and remaining sauce in cups and use as dips. Enjoy!

80) INCREDIBLE SESAME BREADSTICKS

Preparation Time: 10 minutes	**Cooking Time**: 20 minutes	**Servings: 5**

Ingredients:

- ✓ 1 egg white
- ✓ 2 tablespoons almond flour
- ✓ 1 teaspoon Himalayan pink sunflower seeds

Ingredients:

- ✓ 1 tablespoon extra virgin olive oil
- ✓ ½ teaspoon sesame seeds

Directions:

- ❖ P   Preheat the oven to 320 degrees F. Line a baking sheet with baking paper and set aside. Take a bowl and beat the egg whites, add the flour and half of the sunflower seeds and olive oil.

- ❖ Knead until you have a smooth dough. Divide into 4 pieces and roll into breadsticks.

- ❖ Place on prepared sheet and brush with olive oil, sprinkle with remaining sesame seeds and sunflower seeds. Bake for 20 minutes. Serve and enjoy!

81) MEXICAN MEATLOAF

Preparation Time: 15 minutes	**Cooking Time**: 50 minutes	**Servings: 10**

Ingredients:

- ✓ 2 tablespoons of olive oil
- ✓ ½ cup diced onion
- ✓ 1 medium carrot, diced or grated thickly
- ✓ 1 celery stalk, diced
- ✓ 1 garlic clove, minced
- ✓ 1 lb (454 g) ground beef
- ✓ 6 ounces (170 g) of soft Mexican chorizo, removed from the casing and crumbled

Ingredients:

- ✓ 2 jalapeño peppers, diced
- ✓ ¾ teaspoon salt
- ✓ ¼ teaspoon freshly ground black pepper
- ✓ ¼ teaspoon cayenne pepper
- ✓ ½ teaspoon of ground cumin
- ✓ 2 eggs, well beaten
- ✓ ½ cup unseasoned breadcrumbs

Directions:

- ❖ Preheat the oven to 375ºF (190ºC).
- ❖ In a skillet, heat the oil over medium-high heat. Add the onion, carrot, celery, and garlic. Cook, stirring often, until vegetables are soft, about 8 minutes. Set aside until cool enough to handle.
- ❖ In a large bowl, combine sautéed vegetables, ground beef, chorizo and diced jalapeños.

- ❖ In a medium bowl, combine the salt, pepper, cayenne, cumin and eggs. Mix well with a fork and pour over the mixed meats. Add the bread crumbs and mix well with clean hands. (You may want to remove the rings first).
- ❖ Place mixture in a 9-by-13-inch baking dish and insert a meat thermometer in the center. Bake 40 to 45 minutes, or until internal temperature is 160ºF (71ºC). Remove from oven and carefully pour off accumulated cooking juices.

82) PIZZA WITH BEEF, PEPPER AND TOMATO

Preparation Time: 10 minutes	**Cooking Time**: 40 minutes	**Servings: 6-8**

Ingredients:

- ✓ 1 pound (454 g) extra-lean ground sirloin
- ✓ 1 medium onion, thinly sliced
- ✓ 1 or 2 red, yellow or orange peppers, sliced
- ✓ 2 garlic cloves, minced

Ingredients:

- ✓ 1 (14½-ounce / 411-g) can no salt added diced tomatoes
- ✓ Italian seasonings, if necessary
- ✓ 8 ounces (227 g) of 2% chopped mozzarella cheese

Directions:

- ❖ Preheat the oven to 425ºF (220ºC).
- ❖ Heat a large nonstick skillet over medium-high heat. Add ground beef, cook 3 minutes, lower heat to medium. Add the onions, peppers and garlic. Continue cooking for another 5 minutes, or until beef is completely browned and onions are soft.

- ❖ Add the tomatoes and seasonings, and cook another 8-10 minutes to thicken the sauce.
- ❖ Place the ground beef mixture in the bottom of a large shallow glass dish (such as a 1½-quart oval or round Corningware baking dish). Top with shredded mozzarella cheese and bake for 20-25 minutes, or until lightly browned.

83) GRILLED ROMAN STEAK SALAD

Preparation Time: 15 minutes	**Cooking Time**: 10 minutes	**Servings**: 4

Ingredients:

- ✓ 2 boneless New York strip steaks (about 10 ounces / 283 g each)
- ✓ 1 garlic clove, cut in half
- ✓ Salt-free steak seasoning (or mix your own with 1 teaspoon ground black pepper, paprika, garlic powder, onion powder, cayenne pepper, and ¼ teaspoon cilantro)

Ingredients:

- ✓ 4 cups romaine lettuce, cut into 1-inch wide strips
- ✓ 2 ripe pears, sliced
- ✓ Blue cheese crumble (optional)
- ✓ French Vinaigrette, for serving

Directions:

- ❖ Pat the steaks dry with a paper towel. Rub with the chopped garlic clove. Then toss them in the seasoning mixture. Grill the steaks over medium-high heat for about 5 minutes per side, or to the degree you prefer.

- ❖ Slice steaks into 1/2-inch wide strips. Place on top of lettuce; add pear slices and blue cheese (if desired), and drizzle with French vinaigrette.

84) ROLLS OF BEEF LETTUCE AND VEGETABLES

Preparation Time: 20 minutes	**Cooking Time**: 10 minutes	**Servings**: 4

Ingredients:

- ✓ 1 pound (454 g) extra-lean ground sirloin
- ✓ 1 cup diced onions, frozen or fresh
- ✓ 1 cup of red, yellow or orange bell pepper strips, frozen or fresh
- ✓ 1 teaspoon of chili powder
- ✓ 1 teaspoon of paprika
- ✓ ½ teaspoon of onion powder
- ✓ ½ teaspoon of garlic powder

Ingredients:

- ✓ A pinch of cayenne pepper, to taste
- ✓ 4 cups of lettuce
- ✓ 1 cup grated carrots
- ✓ 3 tomatoes, cut into pieces
- ✓ 1 cucumber, diced
- ✓ 1½ cups sweet corn
- ✓ 4 ounces (113 g) shredded Monterey Jack cheese

Directions:

- ❖ Heat a large nonstick skillet over medium-high heat. Add ground beef, onions and peppers, cook 3 minutes and lower heat to medium. Stir occasionally while continuing to cook until the meat is completely browned. Lower the heat to medium-low again and add the seasonings.

- ❖ Plate the lettuce and top with carrots, tomatoes, cucumbers and sweet corn. Place the taco meat and then the cheese.

85) MEXICAN PORK CHOPS

Preparation Time: 10 minutes	**Cooking Time**: 10 minutes	**Servings: 4**

Ingredients:

- ✓ 4 butterfly cut pork chops (2 lbs / 907 g)
- ✓ 1 tablespoon of canola oil
- ✓ Spice Blend
- ✓ 2 tablespoons of paprika
- ✓ 2 tablespoons of chili powder
- ✓ 2 tablespoons of brown sugar

Ingredients:

- ✓ 1 tablespoon ground cumin
- ✓ 1 tablespoon ground black pepper
- ✓ 1 tablespoon of ground white pepper
- ✓ 1 to 2 teaspoons of ground cayenne pepper
- ✓ 1 teaspoon ground cinnamon
- ✓ ½ teaspoon salt

Directions:

- ❖ Mix all the ingredients together for the spice rub.

- ❖ Dip the pork chops in the spices, coating both sides. Heat the oil in a skillet over medium-high heat. Place the pork chops in the skillet, reduce the heat to medium, and cook about 4 minutes on each side, until nicely browned.

86) PORK TENDERLOIN WITH FRUIT

Preparation Time: 10 minutes	**Cooking Time**: 45 minutes	**Servings: 4**

- ✓ 1-pound (454 g) pork tenderloin
- ✓ ½ cup unsweetened dried blueberries
- ✓ ½ cup of dried apricots
- ✓ 1 cup of water
- ✓ 1 cup of Marsala wine

- ✓ 1 teaspoon chopped fresh sage
- ✓ 1 teaspoon fresh tarragon chopped
- ✓ ½ teaspoon of salt substitute
- ✓ ½ teaspoon of freshly ground pepper
- ✓ 1 teaspoon of orange zest

- ❖ Preheat the oven to 375ºF (190ºC).
- ❖ Line a baking sheet with aluminum foil. Place the tenderloin on the foil and arrange the blueberries and apricots around the meat.
- ❖ Pour the water and Marsala wine over everything, then season with sage, tarragon, salt and freshly ground pepper, turning the meat once to coat it evenly.

- ❖ Sprinkle orange zest over the fillet, cover with aluminum foil and bake for 45-50 minutes, uncovering the dish for the last 10 minutes.
- ❖ Let the meat rest for 10 minutes before slicing and arranging it on a serving platter with the sprinkled fruit.

87) DIJON BAKED PORK CHOPS

Preparation Time: 5 minutes	**Cooking Time**: 40 minutes	**Servings: 2**

Ingredients:

- ✓ 2 boneless pork chops
- ✓ Canola oil spray
- ✓ ¾ cup of panko breadcrumbs
- ✓ 2 tablespoons of flour
- ✓ 1 teaspoon of paprika

Ingredients:

- ✓ ¼ teaspoon of sage
- ✓ ¼ teaspoon of garlic powder
- ✓ ¼ teaspoon of chili powder
- ✓ 2 tablespoons of Dijon mustard

- ❖ Preheat the oven to 375ºF (190ºC). Trim pork chops from all fat around the edge. Lightly coat a baking sheet with canola oil spray.

- ❖ Mix the bread crumbs, flour and spices in a shallow bowl. Spread mustard on 1 side of each pork chop and press that side firmly into the breadcrumb mixture. Turn the pork chop over and press that side into the crumbs.
- ❖ Place the pork chops in the baking dish with the mustard side up. Bake uncovered for 40 minutes.

88) PORK CHOPS GLAZED WITH PEACH AND MUSTARD

Preparation Time: 10 minutes	**Cooking Time**: 15 minutes	**Servings**: 4

✓ 4 (4-ounce / 113-g) boneless pork chops, ¾-inch thick (trim all visible fat) ✓ 1 (16-ounce / 454-g) can peach slices in extra light syrup, not drained ✓ 2 tablespoons of peach preserves	✓ 2 tablespoons of Dijon mustard ✓ 1 teaspoon of Worcestershire sauce ✓ 1 teaspoon of black pepper

❖ Combine the peaches, preserves, mustard and Worcestershire sauce in a medium bowl. ❖ Heat a large nonstick skillet over medium-high heat until hot.	❖ Season chops with pepper. Add chops to skillet; brown on both sides. ❖ Add peach mixture to skillet; reduce heat to low. Cover; cook 5 minutes. Serve pork chops topped with peach mixture. Garnish with fresh raspberries, if desired.

89) LAMB TAGINE

Preparation Time: 20 minutes	**Cooking Time**: 1.5 hour	**Servings**: 8

✓ 1 teaspoon of smoked paprika ✓ 1 teaspoon ground turmeric ✓ 1 teaspoon ground cinnamon ✓ ½ teaspoon ground ginger ✓ ½ teaspoon Aleppo pepper or red pepper flakes ✓ 2 pounds (907 g) boneless leg of lamb, cut into 2-inch pieces ✓ 3 tablespoons of olive oil	✓ 1 large onion, chopped (about 2 cups) ✓ 4 garlic cloves, minced ✓ 1 cup low-sodium chicken broth ✓ 3 spoons of honey ✓ 1 pound (454 g) carrots, cut into ½ inch pieces ✓ 6 ounces (170 g) of dried apricots

❖ In a large bowl, combine the smoked paprika, turmeric, cinnamon and Aleppo pepper. Add lamb; stir to coat well. ❖ In a large Dutch oven or tagine, heat 1 tablespoon olive oil. Add half the meat and cook, turning occasionally, for 5 minutes, or until evenly browned. Transfer the meat to a plate. Repeat with a second tablespoon of olive oil and the remaining lamb.	❖ Add the remaining 1 tablespoon of olive oil to the pot. Add onion and cook, stirring frequently, for 5 minutes. Add the broth and honey; stir. Return the lamb and accumulated juices to the pot. Add the carrots and apricots. Raise the heat to high and bring to a boil. Reduce the heat to medium-low, cover, and simmer for 1 hour and 15 minutes to 1 hour and 30 minutes, until the meat is tender. ❖ Serve with couscous or rice, or with crusty bread.

90) GRILLED LAMB CHOPS WITH LEMON AND HERBS

Preparation Time: 10 minutes	**Cooking Time**: 12 minutes	**Servings**: 4-6

Ingredients:	Ingredients:
✓ 3 tablespoons of olive oil ✓ Zest and juice of 1 lemon ✓ 2 tablespoons of pomegranate molasses ✓ 1 cup finely chopped fresh mint	✓ ½ cup finely chopped fresh cilantro or parsley ✓ 2 shallots (green onions), finely chopped ✓ 6 lamb chops ✓ Freshly ground black pepper, to taste

❖ In a small bowl, whisk together the olive oil, lemon zest, lemon juice, pomegranate molasses, mint, parsley and shallots until well combined. Place the lamb in a large zippered plastic bag. Add the marinade, seal the bag and massage the marinade into all sides of the chops. Refrigerate for at least 1 hour or up to overnight.	❖ When you are ready to cook, heat a grill to medium. ❖ Remove chops from marinade; discard marinade. Season with pepper, if desired. Grill chops for 10 to 12 minutes, turning once, for medium. Allow to rest for 10 minutes before serving.

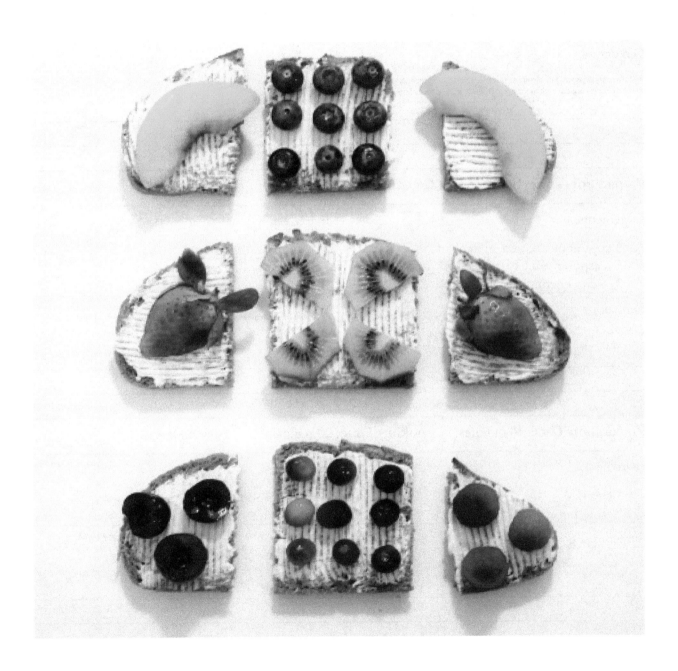

91) ENERGY BITES WITH NUTS WITHOUT COOKING

Preparation Time: 10 minutes	**Cooking Time**:	**Servings: 8 balls**

Ingredients:

- ✓ ¼ cup shredded coconut
- ✓ 1 cup pistachios
- ✓ ½ tablespoon Amaretto liqueur
- ✓ 1 cup almonds

Ingredients:

- ✓ 2 cups pitted dates
- ✓ 2 tablespoons olive oil
- ✓ ¼ cup cocoa powder

Directions:

❖ In a food processor, blend the pistachios, dates, almonds, olive oil, Amaretto liqueur and cocoa powder until well chopped. Make tablespoon-sized balls with the mixture. Roll the balls in the shredded coconut to coat them. Serve chilled.

92) VANILLA APPLE COMPOTE

Preparation Time: 10 minutes	**Cooking Time:** 15 minutes	**Servings: 6**

Ingredients:

- ✓ 3 cups apples, cored and cubed
- ✓ 1 teaspoon vanilla
- ✓ 3/4 cup coconut sugar

Ingredients:

- ✓ 1 cup water
- ✓ 2 tablespoons fresh lime juice

Directions:

❖ Add all ingredients to the inner pot of the Instant Pot and mix well. Seal the pot with the lid and cook on high heat for 15 minutes.

❖ Once done, allow the pressure to release naturally for 10 minutes then release the remaining using the quick release. Remove the lid. Stir and serve.

93) CHOCOLATE RICE

Preparation Time: 10 minutes	**Cooking Time:** 20 minutes	**Servings: 4**

Ingredients:

- ✓ 1 cup rice
- ✓ 1 tablespoon cocoa powder

Ingredients:

- ✓ 2 tablespoons maple syrup
- ✓ 2 cups almond milk

Directions:

❖ Add all ingredients to the inner pot of the robot and mix well. Seal the pot with the lid and cook on high heat for 20 minutes.

❖ Once done, allow the pressure to release naturally for 10 minutes then release the remaining using the quick release. Remove the lid. Stir and serve.

94) MIXTURE OF NUTS, APPLES AND PEARS

Preparation Time: 10 minutes	**Cooking Time**: 10 minutes	**Servings: 4**

Ingredients:	Ingredients:
✓ 2 apples, cored and sliced ✓ 1/2 teaspoon vanilla ✓ 1 cup apple juice	✓ 2 tablespoons walnuts, chopped ✓ 2 apples, cored and sliced
Directions: ❖ Add all ingredients to the inner pot of the Instant Pot and mix well. Seal the pot with the lid and cook on high heat for 10 minutes.	❖ Once done, allow the pressure to release naturally for 10 minutes then release the remaining using the quick release. Remove the lid. Serve and enjoy.

95) PEAR SAUCE

Preparation Time: 10 minutes	**Cooking Time**: 15 minutes	**Servings: 6**

Ingredients:	Ingredients:
✓ 10 pears, sliced ✓ 1 cup apple juice	✓ 1 1/2 teaspoons cinnamon ✓ 1/4 teaspoon nutmeg
Directions: ❖ Add all ingredients to the robot and mix well. Seal the pot with the lid and cook on high heat for 15 minutes. Once done, allow the pressure to release naturally for 10 minutes then release the rest using the quick release.	❖ Remove the lid. Blend the pear mixture using an immersion blender until smooth. Serve and enjoy. ❖ Remove the lid. Blend the pear mixture using an immersion blender until smooth. Serve and enjoy

96) LEMON BLUEBERRY SAUCE

Preparation Time: 10 minutes	**Cooking Time**: 14 minutes	**Servings: 8**

Ingredients:	Ingredients:
✓ 10 ounces fresh blueberries ✓ 3/4 cup Swerve ✓ 1/4 cup water	✓ 1 teaspoon lemon zest ✓ 1 teaspoon vanilla extract
Directions: ❖ Add the blueberries and water to the robot. Seal the pot with the lid and cook on high heat for 1 minute. Once done, allow the pressure to release naturally for 10 minutes then release the rest using the quick release.	❖ • Remove the lid. Set the pot to sauté mode. Add remaining ingredients and cook for 2-3 minutes. Pour into a container and store in the refrigerator

97) BAKED APPLES WITH RAISINS AND PECANS

Preparation Time: 10 minutes	**Cooking Time:** 4 minutes	**Servings: 6**

Ingredients:

- ✓ 6 apples, cored and cut into wedges
- ✓ 1 cup red wine
- ✓ 1/4 cup pecans, chopped
- ✓ 1/4 cup raisins

Ingredients:

- ✓ 1/4 teaspoon nutmeg
- ✓ 1 teaspoon cinnamon
- ✓ 1/3 cup honey

Directions:

❖ Add all ingredients to the robot and mix well. Seal the pot with the lid and cook on high heat for 4 minutes.

❖ Once done, allow the pressure to release naturally for 10 minutes then release the remaining using the quick release. Remove the lid. Stir well and serve.

---

98) MEDITERRANEAN BAKED APPLES

Preparation Time:	**Cooking Time:** 25 minutes	**Servings: 4**

Ingredients:

- ✓ 1.5 lbs. apples, peeled and sliced
- ✓ Juice of ½ lemon

Ingredients:

- ✓ A pinch of cinnamon

Directions:

❖ Preheat oven to 2500F. Line a baking sheet with parchment paper and set aside. In a medium bowl, toss apples with lemon juice and cinnamon.

❖ Place apples on the baking sheet lined with parchment paper. Bake for 25 minutes until crispy.

---

99) MELON AND CUCUMBER SMOOTHIE

Preparation Time:	**Cooking Time:** 5 minutes	**Servings: 2**

Ingredients:

- ✓ ½ cucumber
- ✓ 2 melon slices
- ✓ 2 tablespoons lemon juice

Ingredients:

- ✓ 1 pear, peeled and sliced
- ✓ 3 fresh mint leaves
- ✓ ½ cup almond milk

Directions:

❖ Place all ingredients in a blender. Blend until smooth. Pour into a glass container and let cool in the refrigerator for at least 30 minutes.

100) YOGURT POPS WITH ROASTED BERRIES AND HONEY

Preparation Time:	Cooking Time: 15 minutes	Servings: 8

Ingredients:

- ✓ 12 ounces mixed berries
- ✓ A pinch of sea salt
- ✓ 2 tablespoons honey

Ingredients:

- ✓ 2 cups whole
- ✓ Greek yogurt
- ✓ ½ small lemon, juice

Directions:

- ❖ Preheat the oven to 3500F. Line a baking sheet with baking paper and set aside. In a medium bowl, mix berries with sea salt and honey. Pour the berries onto the prepared baking sheet. Roast for 30 minutes, stirring halfway through.

- ❖ While the fruit roasts, whisk together the Greek yogurt and lemon juice. Add honey to taste, if desired. Once the berries are done, chill for at least ten minutes. Fold the berries into the yogurt mixture. Pour into popsicle molds and let freeze for at least 8 hours. Serve chilled.

101) SUMMER FRUIT SALAD

Preparation Time:	Cooking Time: 5 minutes	Servings: 6

Ingredients:

- ✓ 1 pound strawberries, hulled and thinly sliced
- ✓ 3 medium peaches, thinly sliced
- ✓ 6 ounces blueberries
- ✓ 1 tablespoon fresh mint, chopped

Ingredients:

- ✓ 2 tablespoons lemon juice
- ✓ 1 tablespoon honey
- ✓ 2 teaspoons balsamic vinegar

Directions:

- ❖ In a salad bowl, combine all ingredients. Gently stir to coat all ingredients. Chill for at least 30 minutes before serving.

102) CANTUCCI TOSCANI

Preparation Time: 1 hour 25 minutes	Cooking Time:	Servings: 20 cantucci

Ingredients:

- ✓ Zest of 1 lemon
- ✓ 3/4 cup slivered almonds
- ✓ 2 cups flour
- ✓ 3/4 cup sugar
- ✓ 1 teaspoon baking powder

Ingredients:

- ✓ ¼ teaspoon salt
- ✓ 3 eggs
- ✓ 1 teaspoon olive oil
- ✓ 2 tablespoons Amaretto liqueur

Directions:

- ❖ Preheat oven to 280°F. Combine the flour, baking powder, sugar, lemon zest, salt and almonds in a bowl and mix well. In another bowl, beat the eggs and amaretto liqueur.

- ❖ Pour into the flour mixture and stir to combine. Grease a baking sheet with olive oil and spread the dough. Bake for 40-45 minutes. Remove from oven, let cool for a few minutes and cut diagonally into slices about 1/2 inch thick.
- ❖ Place the pieces back on the sheet, cut sides up, and bake for another 20 minutes. Allow to cool before serving.

103) MAPLE GRILLED PINEAPPLE

Preparation Time: 10 minutes	Cooking Time:	Servings: 4

Ingredients:

- ✓ 1 tablespoon maple syrup
- ✓ 1 pineapple, peeled and cut into wedges

Ingredients:

- ✓ ½ teaspoon cinnamon powder

Directions:

❖ Preheat a grill over high heat. Place fruit in a bowl and drizzle with maple syrup; sprinkle with ground cinnamon.

❖ Grill for about 7-8 minutes, turning occasionally until fruit cracks slightly. Serve.

104) TRADITIONAL GREEK DUMPLINGS WITH HONEY AND PISTACHIOS

Preparation Time: 25 minutes	Cooking Time:	Servings: 4

Ingredients:

- ✓ ½ cup warm milk
- ✓ 2 cups flour
- ✓ 2 eggs, beaten
- ✓ 1 teaspoon sugar
- ✓ 1 ½ oz active dry yeast
- ✓ 1 cup warm water

Ingredients:

- ✓ ½ teaspoon vanilla extract
- ✓ 1 teaspoon cinnamon
- ✓ 1 orange, peeled
- ✓ 1 cup vegetable oil
- ✓ 4 tablespoons honey
- ✓ 2 tablespoons pistachios, chopped

Directions:

❖ In a bowl, sift the flour and combine with the cinnamon and orange zest. In another bowl, mix the sugar, yeast and ½ cup warm water. Let sit until the yeast dissolves.

❖ Stir in the milk, vanilla extract and flour mixture. Beat with an electric mixer for 1-2 minutes until smooth. Cover the bowl with plastic wrap and let rise in a warm place for at least 1 hour. Pour the vegetable oil into a deep skillet or wok to come halfway up the sides and heat the oil. Add more oil if needed.

❖ Using a teaspoon, form balls, one by one, and drop them into the hot oil one by one. Fry the balls on all sides, until golden brown. Remove them with a slotted spoon onto paper towels to absorb excess grease. Repeat the process until the dough is used up. Drizzle with honey and sprinkle with pistachios to serve.

105) SPICY STUFFED APPLES

Preparation Time: 55 minutes	Cooking Time:	Servings: 4

Ingredients:

- ✓ 2 tablespoons brown sugar
- ✓ 4 apples, core
- ✓ ¼ cup chopped pecans

Ingredients:

- ✓ 1 teaspoon cinnamon powder
- ✓ ¼ teaspoon nutmeg powder
- ✓ ¼ teaspoon ginger powder

Directions:

❖ Preheat oven to 375 F. Arrange apples cut side up on a baking sheet. Combine the pecans, cinnamon, brown sugar and nutmeg in a bowl. Pour the mixture into the apples and bake for 35-40 minutes until golden brown. Serve immediately.

106) APPLE DATE BLEND

Preparation Time: 10 minutes	**Cooking Time**: 15 minutes	**Servings: 4**

Ingredients:	Ingredients:
✓ 4 apples, cored and cut into pieces ✓ 1 teaspoon vanilla ✓ 1 teaspoon cinnamon	✓ 1/2 cup pitted dates ✓ 1 1/2 cups apple juice
Directions: ❖ Add all ingredients to the inner pot of the robot and mix well. Seal the pot with the lid and cook on high heat for 15 minutes.	❖ Once done, allow the pressure to release naturally for 10 minutes then release the remaining using the quick release. Remove the lid. Stir and serve.

107) SPECIAL COCOA BROWNIE BOMBS

Preparation Time: 15 minutes	**Cooking Time:** 25 minutes	**Servings: 12**

Ingredients:	Ingredients:
✓ 2 tablespoons grass-fed almond butter ✓ 1 whole egg ✓ 2 teaspoons vanilla extract ✓ ¼ teaspoon baking powder	✓ 1/3 cup heavy cream ✓ 3/4 cup almond butter ✓ ¼ cup cocoa powder ✓ A pinch of sunflower seeds
Directions: ❖ Crack eggs and beat with a whisk until smooth. Add all the wet ingredients and mix well. Make the batter by mixing all the dry ingredients and sifting in the wet ingredients.	❖ Pour into a greased baking dish. Bake for 25 minutes at 350 degrees F or until a toothpick inserted in the center comes out clean. Let cool, cut into slices and serve.

108)	MINI MINT HAPPINESS	
Preparation Time: 45 minutes	**Cooking Time:** 2 hours	**Servings: 12**

Ingredients:	Ingredients:
✓ 2 teaspoons vanilla extract ✓ 1 ½ cups coconut oil ✓ 1 ¼ cups almond butter with sunflower seeds ✓ ½ cup dried parsley	✓ 1 teaspoon peppermint extract ✓ A pinch of sunflower seeds 1 cup dark chocolate chips ✓ Stevia to taste

Directions:

❖ Melt together the coconut oil and dark chocolate chips in a double boiler. Take a food processor, add in all the ingredients and pulse until smooth. Pour into round molds. Allow to freeze.

109)	GENEROUS MAPLE AND PECAN BITES	
Preparation Time: 10 minutes	**Cooking Time:** 25 minutes + freezing	**Servings: 12**

Ingredients:	Ingredients:
✓ 1 cup almond flour ✓ ½ cup coconut oil ✓ ½ cup flaxseed meal ✓ ½ cup unsweetened chocolate chips	✓ 2 cups pecans, chopped ✓ ½ cup unsweetened maple syrup ✓ 20-25 drops Stevia

Directions: ❖ Take a baking sheet and sprinkle pecans on top. Bake at 350 degrees F until aromatic. This usually takes about 6 to 8 minutes. Meanwhile, sift together all the dry ingredients. Add the toasted pecans to the mix and mix well.	❖ Add the coconut oil and maple syrup. Mix to make a thick, sticky mixture. Take a loaf pan lined with parchment paper and pour the mixture into it. Bake for about 18 minutes. Cut into slices and serve.

110)	FANTASTIC BROWNIE MUFFINS	
Preparation Time: 10 minutes	**Cooking Time:** 35 minutes	**Servings: 5**

Ingredients:	Ingredients:
✓ 1 cup golden flaxseed meal ✓ ¼ cup cocoa powder ✓ 1 tablespoon cinnamon ✓ ½ tablespoon baking powder ✓ ½ teaspoon sunflower seeds ✓ 1 large whole egg	✓ 2 tablespoons coconut oil ✓ ¼ cup unsweetened caramel syrup ✓ ½ cup pumpkin puree ✓ 1 teaspoon vanilla extract ✓ 1 teaspoon apple cider vinegar ✓ ¼ cup almonds, shelled

Directions: ❖ Preheat oven to 350 degrees F. Take a bowl and add all of the listed ingredients and mix well. Take the desired number of muffin pans and line them up with paper liners.	❖ Spoon the batter into the muffin pans, filling them up to about 1/4 of the liner. Sprinkle a few almonds on top. Place them in your oven and bake for 15 minutes. Serve warm.

111) SIMPLE GINGERBREAD MUFFINS

Preparation Time: 5 minutes	**Cooking Time**: 30 minutes	**Servings: 12**

Ingredients:

- ✓ 1 tablespoon ground flaxseed
- ✓ 6 tablespoons coconut almond milk
- ✓ 1 tablespoon apple cider vinegar
- ✓ ½ cup peanut almond butter

Ingredients:

- ✓ 2 tablespoons gingerbread spice blend
- ✓ 1 teaspoon baking powder
- ✓ 1 teaspoon vanilla extract
- ✓ 2 tablespoons Swerve

Directions:

- ❖ Preheat the oven to 350 degrees F. Take a bowl and add the flax seeds, sweetener, sunflower seeds, vanilla, spices and your non-dairy almond milk. Set it aside for a bit.

- ❖ Add the peanut almond butter, baking powder and continue to mix until well combined. Stir in the peanut almond butter and baking powder. Mix well.
- ❖ Spoon the mixture into muffin liners. Bake for 30 minutes. Let them cool and enjoy!

112) NUTMEG NOUGATS

Preparation Time: 10 minutes	**Cooking Time**: 5 minutes + 30 minutes freezing time	**Servings: 12**

Ingredients:

- ✓ 1 cup coconut, shredded
- ✓ 1 cup low-fat cream

Ingredients:

- ✓ 1 cup cashew almond butter
- ✓ ½ teaspoon nutmeg powder

Directions:

- ❖ Melt the cashew and almond butter in a double boiler. Add nutmeg and cream cheese. Remove from heat. Allow to cool a bit. Keep in the refrigerator for at least 30 minutes.

- ❖ Remove from refrigerator and make small balls. Coat with shredded coconut. Let cool for 2 hours and then serve.

113) RASPBERRY SUPREME CHOCOLATE BOMBS

Preparation Time: 10 minutes	**Cooking Time**: /[MOU2] Freezing Time: 1 hour	**Servings: 6**

Ingredients:

- ✓ ½ cocoa almond butter
- ✓ ½ coconut manna
- ✓ 4 tablespoons coconut milk powder

Ingredients:

- ✓ 3 tablespoons granulated stevia
- ✓ ¼ cup dried and crushed raspberries, frozen

Directions:

- ❖ Prepare double boiler over medium heat and melt cocoa almond butter and coconut manna. Stir in the vanilla extract. Take another pot and add the coconut powder and sugar substitute.

- ❖ Stir the coconut mixture into the cocoa butter, 1 tablespoon at a time, making sure to keep stirring after each addition. Add the crushed dried raspberries. Mix well and distribute into muffin pans. Chill for 60 minutes and enjoy!

114) CASHEW AND ALMOND BUTTER

Preparation Time: 5 minutes	Cooking Time:	Servings: 1
✓ 1 cup almonds, blanched ✓ 1/3 cup cashews ✓ 2 tablespoons coconut oil	✓ Sunflower seeds as needed ✓ ½ teaspoon cinnamon	
Directions: ❖ Preheat oven to 350 degrees F. Bake almonds and cashews for 12 minutes. Allow them to cool.	❖ Transfer to food processor and add remaining ingredients. Add oil and continue blending until smooth. Serve and enjoy!	

115) ELEGANT CRANBERRY MUFFINS

Preparation Time: 10 minutes	Cooking Time: 20 minutes	Servings: 24 muffins
✓ 2 cups almond flour ✓ 2 teaspoons baking soda ✓ ¼ cup avocado oil ✓ 1 whole egg ✓ ¾ cup almond milk	✓ ½ cup erythritol ✓ ½ cup applesauce ✓ Zest of 1 orange ✓ 2 teaspoons cinnamon powder ✓ 2 cups fresh blueberries	
Directions: ❖ Preheat oven to 350 degrees F. Line muffin pan with paper cups and set aside. Add the flour, baking soda and set aside. Take another bowl and whisk the remaining ingredients and add the flour, mix well.	❖ Pour the batter into the prepared muffin pan and bake for 20 minutes. Once done, let cool for 10 minutes. Serve and enjoy!	

116) FASHIONABLE CHOCOLATE PARFAIT

Preparation Time: 2 hours	Cooking Time:	Servings: 4
✓ 2 tablespoons cocoa powder ✓ 1 cup almond milk ✓ 1 tablespoon chia seeds	✓ Pinch sunflower seeds ✓ ½ teaspoon vanilla extract	
❖ Take a bowl and add the cocoa powder, almond milk, chia seeds, vanilla extract and mix. Transfer to a dessert glass and refrigerate for 2 hours. Serve and enjoy!		

117) MESMERIZING AVOCADO AND CHOCOLATE PUDDING

Preparation Time: 30 minutes	Cooking Time:	Servings: 2
✓ 1 avocado, chopped ✓ 1 tablespoon natural sweetener such as stevia ✓ 2 ounces cream cheese, room temperature	✓ ¼ teaspoon vanilla extract ✓ 4 tablespoons cocoa powder, unsweetened	
Directions: ❖ Blend listed ingredients in blender until smooth. Divide the mixture between dessert bowls, chill for 30 minutes. Serve and enjoy!		

118) HEALTHY BERRY TART

Preparation Time: 10 minutes	**Cooking Time**: 2 hours 30 minutes	**Servings**: 8

Ingredients:	Ingredients:
✓ 1 ¼ cups almond flour	✓ ¼ cup low-fat milk
✓ 1 cup coconut sugar	✓ 2 tablespoons olive oil
✓ 1 teaspoon baking powder	✓ 2 cups raspberries
✓ ½ teaspoon cinnamon powder	✓ 2 cups blueberries
✓ 1 whole egg	

Directions:

❖ Take a bowl and add the almond flour, coconut sugar, baking powder and cinnamon. Mix well. Take another bowl and add the egg, milk, oil,

119) SPICED POPCORN

Preparation Time: 2 minutes	**Cooking Time**:	**Servings**: 4

Ingredients:	Ingredients:
✓ ½ teaspoon of chili powder	✓ ⅛ teaspoon of cayenne
✓ ⅛ teaspoon of garlic powder without salt	✓ 8 cups of air popped popcorn
✓ ⅛ teaspoon of paprika	

Directions:	❖ Place popcorn in a large bowl and toss with the spice mixture. Serve immediately or store in an airtight container for up to 2 days.
❖ In a small bowl, combine the chili powder, garlic powder, paprika and cayenne.	

120) BAKED TORTILLA CHIPS WITH LIME

Preparation Time: 5 minutes	**Cooking Time**: 25 minutes	**Servings**: 6

Ingredients:	Ingredients:
✓ 4 teaspoons of lime juice	✓ 12 corn tortillas (6 inches)
✓ 2 teaspoons of canola oil	✓ Kitchen spray
✓ ½ teaspoon of ground cumin	

Directions:	❖ Arrange the tortilla pieces in a single layer on the prepared baking sheets. Bake in the preheated oven, rotating the pans every 10 minutes, until the chips are golden brown and potato chip, about 25 minutes.
❖ Preheat oven to 400°F (205°C). Spray two large baking sheets with cooking spray.	
❖ In a small bowl, mix together the lime juice, canola oil and cumin. Brush each tortilla on both sides with the mixture and cut into 6 wedges	

BOOK 2: DASH DIET FOR HIM

Chapter 1. BREAKFAST AND SNACKS

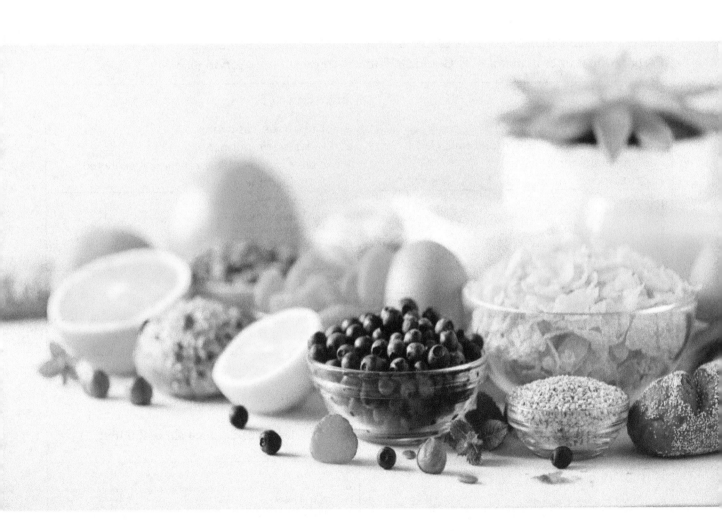

121)   BANANA STEEL OATS

Preparation Time: 10 minutes	**Cooking Time:** 15 minutes	**Servings: 3**

Ingredients:

- ✓ 1 small banana
- ✓ 1 cup almond milk
- ✓ ¼ teaspoon cinnamon, ground

Ingredients:

- ✓ ½ cup rolled oats
- ✓ 1 tablespoon honey

Directions:

- ❖ Take a casserole dish and add half of the banana, whisk in almond milk, ground cinnamon.
- ❖ Season with the sunflower seeds. Stir until the banana is well mashed, bring the mixture to a boil and stir in the oats.

- ❖ Reduce heat to medium-low and simmer for 5-7 minutes until oats are tender.
- ❖ Dice the remaining half of the banana and place on top of the oatmeal. Enjoy!

122)   PINEAPPLE OATMEAL

Preparation Time: 10 minutes	**Cooking Time:** 4-8 hours	**Servings: 5**

Ingredients:

- ✓ 1 cup steel-cut oats
- ✓ 4 cups unsweetened almond milk
- ✓ 2 medium apples, sliced
- ✓ 1 teaspoon coconut oil

Ingredients:

- ✓ 1 teaspoon cinnamon
- ✓ ¼ teaspoon nutmeg
- ✓ 2 tablespoons maple syrup, unsweetened
- ✓ A trickle of lemon juice

Directions:

- ❖ Add the listed ingredients to a pot and mix well.
- ❖ Cook on very low heat for 8 hours or on high heat for 4 hours.

- ❖ Stir gently. Add desired toppings. Serve and enjoy!
- ❖ Store in the refrigerator for later use; be sure to add a splash of almond milk after reheating for added flavor.

123)   CRISPY FLAX AND ALMOND CRACKERS

Preparation Time: 15 minutes	**Cooking Time:** 60 minutes	**Servings: 20-24 crackers**

Ingredients:

- ✓ ½ cup ground flaxseed
- ✓ ½ cup almond flour
- ✓ 1 tablespoon coconut flour
- ✓ 2 tablespoons shelled hemp seeds

Ingredients:

- ✓ ¼ teaspoon sunflower seeds
- ✓ 1 egg white
- ✓ 2 tablespoons unsalted almond butter, melted

Directions:

- ❖ Preheat oven to 300 degrees F.
- ❖ Line a baking sheet with baking paper, set aside.
- ❖ Add flax, almonds, coconut flour, hemp seeds to a bowl and mix.

- ❖ Add egg whites and melted almond butter, mix until combined.
- ❖ Transfer dough to a sheet of parchment paper and cover with another sheet of paper.
- ❖ Roll out dough. Cut into crackers and bake for 60 minutes. Let them cool and enjoy!

124)	COOL MUSHROOM MUNCHIES	
Preparation Time: 5 minutes	**Cooking Time**: 10 minutes	**Servings**: 2

Ingredients:

- ✓ 4 caps Portobello mushrooms
- ✓ 3 tablespoons coconut aminos
- ✓ 2 tablespoons sesame oil

Ingredients:

- ✓ 1 tablespoon fresh ginger, minced
- ✓ 1 small clove garlic, minced

Directions:

- ❖ Set the oven to low, keeping the rack 6 inches from the heat source.
- ❖ Wash the mushrooms under cold water and transfer them to a baking sheet (top side down).

- ❖ Take a bowl and mix the sesame oil, garlic, coconut amino acid, ginger and pour the mixture over the tops of the mushrooms.
- ❖ Cook for 10 minutes. Serve and enjoy!

125)	DELICIOUS BOWL OF QUINOA WITH BERRIES	
Preparation Time: 5 minutes	**Cooking Time**: 15 minutes	**Servings**: 4

Ingredients:

- ✓ 1 cup quinoa
- ✓ 2 cups water
- ✓ 1 2-inch piece of cinnamon stick
- ✓ 2-3 tablespoons maple syrup Flavorful toppings
- ✓ ½ cup blueberries, raspberries or strawberries

Ingredients:

- ✓ 2 tablespoons raisins
- ✓ 1 teaspoon lime
- ✓ ¼ teaspoon nutmeg, grated
- ✓ 3 tablespoons whipped coconut cream
- ✓ 2 tablespoons cashews, chopped

Directions:

- ❖ Take a metal strainer and pass your grains through it to filter them well.
- ❖ Rinse the grains well under cold water.
- ❖ Take a medium sized saucepan and pour in the water.
- ❖ Add the strained grains and bring it to a boil.
- ❖ Add the cinnamon sticks and cover the saucepan.

- ❖ Lower the heat and let the mixture simmer for 15 minutes to allow the grains to absorb the liquid.
- ❖ Remove the heat and stir the mixture with a fork.
- ❖ Add maple syrup if you want additional flavor.
- ❖ Also, if you want to make things a little more interesting, just add any of the above ingredients.

126)	BOWL OF QUINOA AND CINNAMON	
Preparation Time: 10 minutes	**Cooking Time**: 15 minutes	**Servings**: 2

Ingredients:

- ✓ 1 cup uncooked quinoa
- ✓ 1½ cups water
- ✓ ½ teaspoon cinnamon powder

Ingredients:

- ✓ ½ teaspoon sunflower seeds
- ✓ A drizzle of almond/coconut milk to serve

- ❖ Rinse the quinoa well under water.
- ❖ Take a medium sized saucepan and add the quinoa, water, cinnamon and seeds.
- ❖ Stir and place over medium-high heat. Bring the mix to a boil.

- ❖ Reduce the heat to low and simmer for 10 minutes.
- ❖ Once cooked, remove from heat and allow to cool.
- ❖ Serve with a drizzle of almond or coconut milk. Enjoy!

127)	AMAZING AND HEALTHY BOWL OF GRANOLA	
Preparation Time: 5 minutes	**Cooking Time**: 25 minutes	**Servings**: 6

Ingredients:

- ✓ 1 ounce oatmeal Porridge
- ✓ 2 teaspoons maple syrup Cooking spray if needed
- ✓ 4 medium bananas
- ✓ 4 jars of Fromage Frais layered caramel
- ✓ 5 ounces fresh fruit salad, such as strawberries, blueberries and raspberries

Ingredients:

- ✓ ¼ ounce pumpkin seeds
- ✓ ¼ ounce sunflower seeds
- ✓ ¼ ounce dried chia seeds
- ✓ ¼ ounce dried coconut

Directions:

- ❖ Preheat oven to 300 degrees F.
- ❖ Take a baking sheet and line with baking paper.
- ❖ Take a large bowl and add oats, maple syrup and seeds.
- ❖ Spread the mix on a baking sheet.

- ❖ Drizzle coconut oil on top and bake for 20 minutes, making sure to keep stirring occasionally.
- ❖ Sprinkle with coconut after the first 15 minutes. Remove from oven and allow to cool.
- ❖ Take a bowl and layer sliced bananas on top of the Fromage Fraise.
- ❖ Spread the cooled granola mix on top and serve with a berry garnish. Enjoy!

128)	BOWL OF QUINOA AND DATES	
Preparation Time: 10 minutes	**Cooking Time**: 15 minutes	**Servings**: 2

Ingredients:

- ✓ 1 date, pitted and finely chopped
- ✓ ½ cup red quinoa, dried
- ✓ 1 cup unsweetened almond milk

Ingredients:

- ✓ 1/8 teaspoon vanilla extract
- ✓ ¼ cup fresh strawberries, hulled and sliced
- ✓ 1/8 teaspoon cinnamon powder

Directions:

- ❖ Take a skillet and place it over low heat.

- ❖ Add the quinoa, almond milk, cinnamon, and vanilla and cook for about 15 minutes,
- ❖ making sure to keep stirring occasionally.
- ❖ Garnish with the strawberries and enjoy!

129)	PUMPKIN OATS	
Preparation Time: 5 minutes	**Cooking Time**: 8 minutes	**Servings**: 3

Ingredients:

- ✓ 1 cup quick-cooking rolled oats
- ✓ ¾ cup almond milk
- ✓ ½ cup canned pumpkin puree

Ingredients:

- ✓ ¼ teaspoon pumpkin spice
- ✓ 1 teaspoon cinnamon powder

Directions:

- ❖ Take a microwave safe bowl and add the oats, almond milk and microwave for 1-2 minutes.
- ❖ Add more almond milk if needed to reach desired consistency.

- ❖ Cook for an additional 30 seconds.
- ❖ Stir in the pumpkin puree, pumpkin pie spice and ground cinnamon. Heat gently and enjoy!

130) ENERGY-RICH OATMEAL

Preparation Time: 10-15 minutes	**Cooking Time**: 5 minutes	**Servings**: 2

Ingredients:

- ¼ cup quick-cooking oats
- ¼ cup almond milk
- 2 tablespoons low-fat Greek yogurt

Ingredients:

- ¼ cup banana, mashed
- 2-1/4 tablespoons flaxseed meal

Directions:

- Whisk all ingredients together in a bowl.

- Transfer the bowl to your refrigerator and let sit for 15 minutes.
- Serve and enjoy!

131) MOUTH WATERING CHICKEN PORRIDGE

Preparation Time: 1 hour	**Cooking Time**: 10-20 minutes	**Servings**: 4

Ingredients:

- 1 cup jasmine rice
- 1 pound steamed/cooked chicken thighs
- 5 cups chicken broth

Ingredients:

- 4 cups water
- 1 ½ cups fresh ginger Green onions Roasted cashews

Directions:

- Put the rice in the refrigerator and let it cool 1 hour before cooking.
- Take out the rice and add it to your Robot.
- Pour in the chicken broth and water.
- Close the lid and cook in PORRIDGE mode, using your default settings and parameters.

- Release pressure naturally in 10 minutes.
- Open the lid. Remove the meat from the chicken thighs and add the meat to the soup.
- Stir well in Sauté mode. Season with a little flavored vinegar and enjoy with a garnish of walnuts and onion.

132) THE "PORRIDGE" OF DECISIVE APPLES

Preparation Time: 10 minutes	**Cooking Time**: 5 minutes	**Servings**: 2

Ingredients:

- 1 large apple, peeled, pitted and grated
- 1 cup unsweetened almond milk
- 1 ½ tablespoons sunflower seeds

Ingredients:

- 1/8 cup fresh blueberries
- ¼ teaspoon fresh vanilla bean extract

Directions:

- Take a large skillet and add the sunflower seeds, vanilla extract, almond milk, apples and stir.

- Place over medium-low heat. Cook for 5 minutes, making sure to keep the mixture stirred. Transfer to a serving bowl. Serve and enjoy

133) CINNAMON AND COCONUT PORRIDGE

Preparation Time: 5 minutes	**Cooking Time:** 5 minutes	**Servings:** 4

Ingredients:

- ✓ 2 cups water
- ✓ 1 cup cream of coconut
- ✓ ½ cup unsweetened dry coconut, shredded
- ✓ 2 tablespoons flaxseed meal

Ingredients:

- ✓ 1 tablespoon almond butter
- ✓ 1 ½ teaspoons stevia
- ✓ 1 teaspoon cinnamon Toppings such as blueberries

Directions:

- ❖ Add the listed ingredients to a small saucepan, stir well.
- ❖ Transfer the pot to the stove and place it over medium-low heat.
- ❖ Bring everything to a slow boil.

- ❖ Stir well and remove from heat.
- ❖ Divide the mixture into equal portions and let them rest for 10 minutes. Top with desired toppings and enjoy!

134) VANILLA SWEET POTATO PORRIDGE

Preparation Time: 10 minutes	**Cooking Time:** 8 hours	**Servings:** 5

Ingredients:

- ✓ 6 sweet potatoes, peeled and cut into
- ✓ 1-inch cubes
- ✓ 1 ½ cups light coconut milk
- ✓ 1 teaspoon cinnamon powder

Ingredients:

- ✓ 1 teaspoon cardamom powder
- ✓ 1 teaspoon pure vanilla extract
- ✓ 1 cup raisins Pinch of salt

Directions:

- ❖ Add the sweet potatoes, coconut milk, vanilla, cardamom and cinnamon to your Slow Cooker.
- ❖ Close the lid and cook on LOW for 8 hours.

- ❖ Open the lid and mash all the mixture using a potato masher to mash the sweet potatoes, mix well.
- ❖ Add the raisins, salt and serve. Serve and enjoy!

135) BANANA OATMEAL VERY NUTRITIOUS

Preparation Time: 15 minutes	**Cooking Time:** 7-9 hours	**Servings:** 4

Ingredients:

- ✓ 1 cup steel-cut oats
- ✓ 1 ripe banana, mashed
- ✓ 2 cups unsweetened almond milk
- ✓ 1 cup water
- ✓ 1 ½ tablespoons honey

Ingredients:

- ✓ ½ teaspoon vanilla extract
- ✓ ¼ cup almonds, chopped
- ✓ 1 teaspoon cinnamon powder
- ✓ ¼ teaspoon nutmeg powder

Directions:

- ❖ Grease the pressure cooker well.
- ❖ Add the listed ingredients to the pressure cooker and stir.

- ❖ Cover with lid and cook on LOW for 7-9 hours. Serve and enjoy!

136)	PERFECT HOMEMADE PICKLED GINGER GARI	
Preparation Time: 40 minutes	**Cooking Time**: 5 minutes	**Servings**: 8

Ingredients:

- ✓ Approximately 8 ounces fresh ginger root, fully peeled
- ✓ 1 teaspoon and extra
- ✓ ½ teaspoon fine sunflower seeds

Ingredients:

- ✓ 1 cup vinegar, rice
- ✓ 1/3 cup sugar, white

Directions:

- ❖ Cut ginger into small pieces and transfer to a bowl.
- ❖ Season with sunflower seeds and stir, let the mixture sit for at least 30 minutes.
- ❖ Take a saucepan and add the sugar and vinegar, heat, bring the mixture to a boil and continue to boil until the sugar has completely dissolved.

- ❖ Pour the liquid over the ginger pieces.
- ❖ Let cool and wait for the water to change color. Enjoy! Alternatively, store in jars and use as needed.

137)	HEALTHY SAUTÉED ZUCCHINI	
Preparation Time: 10 minutes	**Cooking Time**: 10 minutes	**Servings**: 4

Ingredients:

- ✓ 2 heaped tablespoons olive oil
- ✓ 1 medium onion, thinly sliced
- ✓ 2 medium zucchini, cut into thin strips

Ingredients:

- ✓ 2 heaped tablespoons teriyaki sauce, low sodium
- ✓ 1 tablespoon coconut aminos
- ✓ 1 tablespoon sesame seeds, toasted Ground pepper (black) as needed

Directions:

- ❖ Take a skillet and place it on the stove on medium level.
- ❖ Add the onions and stir for 5 minutes.
- ❖ Add the zucchini and stir for 1 more minute.

- ❖ Gently add the sauces along with the sesame seeds.
- ❖ Cook for another 5 minutes until the zucchini is soft.
- ❖ Finally, add the pepper and enjoy!

138)	INCREDIBLE SCRAMBLED TURKEY EGGS	
Preparation Time: 15 minutes	**Cooking Time**: 15 minutes	**Servings**: 2

Ingredients:

- ✓ 1 tablespoon coconut oil
- ✓ 1 medium red bell pepper, diced
- ✓ ½ medium yellow onion, diced
- ✓ ¼ teaspoon chili sauce

Ingredients:

- ✓ 3 large free-range eggs
- ✓ ¼ teaspoon black pepper, freshly ground
- ✓ ¼ teaspoon salt

- ❖ Place a skillet over medium-high heat, add the coconut oil and let it heat up.
- ❖ Add the onions and sauté.
- ❖ Add the turkey and red bell bell pepper.

- ❖ Cook until the turkey is cooked through. Take a bowl and beat the eggs, stir in salt and pepper.
- ❖ Pour the eggs into the pan with the turkey and gently cook and scramble the eggs.
- ❖ Add the hot sauce and enjoy!

139) SPICY SALAMI OMELETTE

Preparation Time: 5 minutes	**Cooking Time**: 20 minutes	**Servings**: 2

Ingredients:

✓ 3 eggs
✓ 7 slices of pepperoni
✓ 1 teaspoon of coconut cream

Ingredients:

✓ Salt and freshly ground black pepper, to taste
✓ 1 tablespoon of butter

Directions:

❖ Take a bowl and beat the eggs with all the remaining ingredients.
❖ Then take a skillet and heat the butter. Pour ¼ of the egg mixture into the pan.

❖ After that, cook for 2 minutes on each side.
❖ Repeat to use the entire batter. Serve hot and enjoy!

140) OMELETTE WITH HERBS AND AVOCADO

Preparation Time: 2 minutes	**Cooking Time**: 10 minutes	**Servings**: 2

Ingredients:

✓ 3 large free-range eggs
✓ ½ medium avocado, sliced

Ingredients:

✓ ½ cup almonds, sliced Salt and pepper to taste

Directions:

❖ Take a non-stick skillet and place it over medium-high heat.
❖ Take a bowl and add the eggs, beat the eggs. Pour into the skillet and cook for 1 minute.

❖ Reduce the heat to low and cook for 4 minutes. Top the omelet with the almonds and avocado.
❖ Sprinkle with salt and pepper and serve. Enjoy!

141) CARROT AND ZUCCHINI OATMEAL

Preparation Time: 10 minutes	**Cooking Time**: 8 hours	**Servings**: 3

Ingredients:

✓ ½ cup steel-cut oats
✓ 1 cup coconut milk
✓ 1 carrot, grated
✓ ¼ cup zucchini, grated

Ingredients:

✓ A pinch of nutmeg
✓ ½ teaspoon cinnamon powder
✓ 2 tablespoons brown sugar
✓ ¼ cup pecans, chopped

Directions:

❖ Grease Slow Cooker pot well.
❖ Add oats, zucchini, milk, carrot, nutmeg, cloves, sugar, cinnamon and mix well.

❖ Place lid on and cook on LOW for 8 hours.
❖ Divide between serving bowls and enjoy!

Chapter 2. LUNCH

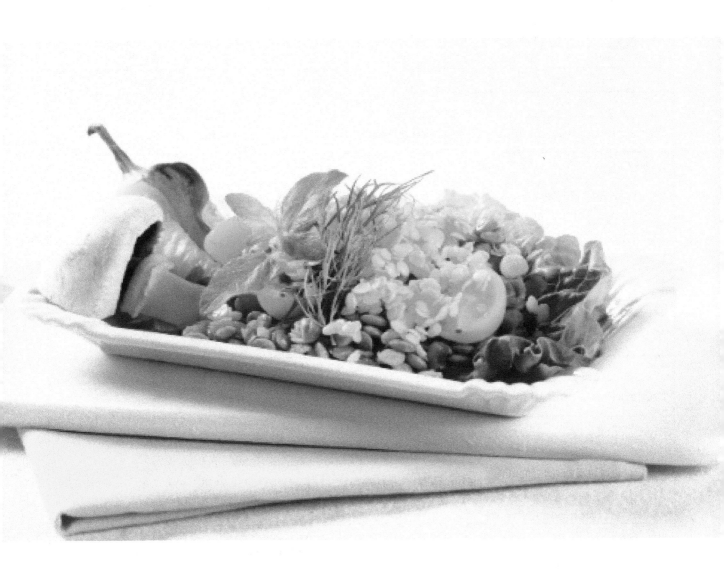

142) FANTASTIC MANGO CHICKEN

Preparation Time: 25 minutes	**Cooking Time:** 10 minutes	**Servings:** 4

Ingredients:

- ✓ 2 medium mangoes, peeled and chopped 10 ounces coconut milk 4 teaspoons vegetable oil 4 teaspoons spicy curry paste 14 ounces boneless,

Ingredients:

- ✓ skinless chicken breast, diced 4 medium shallots 1 large English cucumber, sliced and seeded

Directions:

- ❖ Slice half of the mangoes and add the halves to a bowl. Add the mangoes and almond and coconut milk to a blender and blend until smooth. Keep the mixture aside. Take a large pot and place it on a medium heat, add the oil and let the oil heat up.

- ❖ Add the curry paste and cook for 1 minute until fragrant, add the shallots and chicken to the pot and cook for 5 minutes. Pour in the mango puree and let it heat through. Serve the cooked chicken with the mango puree and cucumbers. Enjoy

143) CHICKEN LIVER STEW

Preparation Time: 10 minutes	**Cooking Time:** Zero	**Servings:** 2

Ingredients:

- ✓ 10 ounces chicken livers
- ✓ 1 ounce onion, chopped

Ingredients:

- ✓ 2 ounces sour cream
- ✓ 1 tablespoon olive oil Sunflower seeds to taste

Directions:

- ❖ Take a frying pan and place it over medium heat.
- ❖ Add the oil and let it heat up.
- ❖ Add the onions and sauté until just golden brown. Add the livers and season with the sunflower seeds.

- ❖ Cook until the livers are halfway cooked.
- ❖ Transfer the mixture to a stew pot.
- ❖ Add the sour cream and cook for 20 minutes. Serve and enjoy!

144) CHICKEN WITH MUSTARD

Preparation Time: 10 minutes	**Cooking Time:** 40 minutes	**Servings:** 2

Ingredients:

- ✓ 2 chicken breasts
- ✓ 1/4 cup chicken broth
- ✓ 2 tablespoons mustard
- ✓ 1 1/2 tablespoons olive oil

Ingredients:

- ✓ 1/2 teaspoon paprika
- ✓ 1/2 teaspoon chili powder
- ✓ 1/2 teaspoon garlic powder

Directions:

- ❖ Take a small bowl and mix the mustard, olive oil, paprika, chicken broth, garlic powder, chicken broth and chili.
- ❖ Add the chicken breast and marinate for 30 minutes.

- ❖ Take a lined baking sheet and arrange the chicken.
- ❖ Bake for 35 minutes at 375 degrees F. Serve and enjoy!

145) THE DELICIOUS TURKEY WRAP

Preparation Time: 10 minutes	**Cooking Time:** 10 minutes	**Servings: 6**

Ingredients:

- ✓ 1 ¼ pounds ground turkey, lean
- ✓ 4 green onions, chopped
- ✓ 1 tablespoon olive oil
- ✓ 1 clove garlic, minced
- ✓ 2 teaspoons chili paste
- ✓ 8 ounces water chestnuts, diced

Ingredients:

- ✓ 3 tablespoons hoisin sauce
- ✓ 2 tablespoons coconut aminos
- ✓ 1 tablespoon rice vinegar
- ✓ 12 almond butter lettuce leaves
- ✓ 1/8 teaspoon sunflower seeds

Directions:

- ❖ Take a skillet and place it over medium heat, add the turkey and garlic to the pan.
- ❖ Heat for 6 minutes until cooked through.
- ❖ Take a bowl and transfer the turkey to it.

- ❖ Add the onions and water chestnuts.
- ❖ Stir in the hoisin sauce, coconut amino acid, vinegar and chili paste.
- ❖ Mix well and transfer to lettuce leaves. Serve and enjoy!

146) ZUCCHINI ZOODLES WITH CHICKEN AND BASIL

Preparation Time: 10 minutes	**Cooking Time:** 10 minutes	**Servings: 3**

Ingredients:

- ✓ 2 chicken fillets, diced
- ✓ 2 tablespoons ghee
- ✓ 1 pound tomatoes, diced
- ✓ ½ cup basil, chopped

Ingredients:

- ✓ ¼ cup almond milk
- ✓ 1 garlic clove, peeled, chopped
- ✓ 1 zucchini, chopped

Directions:

- ❖ Fry the diced chicken in the ghee until no longer pink.
- ❖ Add the tomatoes and season with the sunflower seeds.
- ❖ Simmer and reduce the liquid.

- ❖ Prepare the Zoodles by shredding the zucchini in a food processor.
- ❖ Add the basil, garlic, coconut and almond milk to the chicken and cook for a few minutes.
- ❖ Add half of the Zucchini Zoodles to a bowl and top with the creamy tomato basil chicken. Enjoy!

147) BAKED CHICKEN WITH PARMESAN CHEESE

Preparation Time: 5 minutes	**Cooking Time:** 20 minutes	**Servings: 2**

Ingredients:

- ✓ 2 tablespoons ghee
- ✓ 2 boneless chicken breasts, skinless Pink sunflower seeds Freshly ground black pepper
- ✓ ½ cup mayonnaise, low-fat

Ingredients:

- ✓ ¼ cup Parmesan cheese, grated
- ✓ 1 tablespoon dry Italian seasoning, low-fat, low-sodium
- ✓ ¼ cup crushed pork rind

- ❖ Preheat oven to 425 degrees F. Take a large baking sheet and coat with ghee.
- ❖ Pat the chicken breasts dry and wrap with a towel. Season with sunflower seeds and pepper.
- ❖ Place in the baking dish.

- ❖ Take a small bowl and add the mayonnaise, parmesan cheese and Italian seasoning.
- ❖ Spread mayonnaise mixture evenly over chicken breast. Sprinkle with crushed pork rind.
- ❖ Bake for 20 minutes until the topping is golden brown. Serve and enjoy!

148) CRAZY JAPANESE POTATO AND BEEF CROQUETTES

Preparation Time: 10 minutes	**Cooking Time:** 20 minutes	**Servings: 10**

Ingredients:

- ✓ 3 medium russet potatoes, peeled and chopped
- ✓ 1 tablespoon almond butter
- ✓ 1 tablespoon vegetable oil
- ✓ 3 onions, diced

Ingredients:

- ✓ ¾ pound ground beef
- ✓ 4 teaspoons light coconut aminos All-purpose flour for coating
- ✓ 2 eggs, beaten Panko bread crumbs for coating
- ✓ ½ cup oil for frying

Directions:

- ❖ Take a saucepan and place it over medium-high heat; add the potatoes and sunflower seed water, boil for 16 minutes.
- ❖ Remove the water and place the potatoes in another bowl, add the almond butter and mash the potatoes.
- ❖ Take a frying pan and put it on medium heat, add 1 tablespoon of oil and let it heat up.
- ❖ Add the onions and sauté until tender. Add the beef coconut aminos to the onions.

- ❖ Continue frying until the beef is browned. Mix the beef with the potatoes evenly.
- ❖ Take another skillet and place it over medium heat; add half a cup of oil.
- ❖ Form croquettes with the mashed potato mixture and coat with flour, then egg and finally breadcrumbs.
- ❖ Fry the croquettes until golden brown on all sides. Enjoy!

149) GOLDEN EGGPLANT CHIPS

Preparation Time: 10 minutes	**Cooking Time:** 15 minutes	**Servings: 8**

Ingredients:

- ✓ 2 eggs
- ✓ 2 cups almond flour

Ingredients:

- ✓ 2 tablespoons coconut oil, spray
- ✓ 2 eggplants, peeled and thinly sliced Sunflower seeds and pepper

Directions:

- ❖ Preheat oven to 400 degrees F.
- ❖ Take a bowl and stir in sunflower seeds and black pepper.
- ❖ Take another bowl and beat the eggs until frothy.
- ❖ Dip the eggplant pieces into the eggs.

- ❖ Then coat them with the flour mixture.
- ❖ Add another layer of flour and eggs.
- ❖ Then, take a baking sheet and grease it with coconut oil on top.
- ❖ Bake for about 15 minutes. Serve and enjoy!

150) VERY WILD MUSHROOMS PILAF

Preparation Time: 10 minutes	Cooking Time: 3 hours	Servings: 4

Ingredients:	Ingredients:
✓ 1 cup wild rice ✓ 2 cloves minced garlic ✓ 6 chopped green onions	✓ 2 tablespoons olive oil ✓ ½ pound baby Bella mushrooms ✓ 2 cups water

Directions:	❖ Put the lid on and cook on LOW for 3 hours. ❖ Stir the pilaf and divide between serving plates. Enjoy!
❖ Add the rice, garlic, onion, oil, mushrooms and water to your Slow Cooker. ❖ Stir well until combined.	

151) SPORTS CARROTS FOR KIDS

Preparation Time: 5 minutes	Cooking Time: 5 minutes	Servings: 4

Ingredients:	Ingredients:
✓ 1 pound baby carrots ✓ 1 cup water	✓ 1 tablespoon clarified ghee ✓ 1 tablespoon chopped fresh mint leaves Flavored sea vinegar, if needed

Directions:	❖ Return the insert to the pot and set the pot to Sauté mode. Add the clarified butter and let it melt. ❖ Add the mint and sauté for 30 seconds. Add the carrots to the insert and sauté well. ❖ Remove them and sprinkle some of the flavored vinegar on top. Enjoy
❖ Place a steamer basket on top of your pot and add the carrots. Add the water. ❖ Close the lid and cook at HIGH pressure for 2 minutes. Make a quick release. ❖ Pass the carrots through a strainer and drain. Clean the insert.	

152) GARDEN SALAD

Preparation Time: 5 minutes	Cooking Time: 20 minutes	Servings: 6

Ingredients:	Ingredients:
✓ 1 pound raw peanuts in shell ✓ 1 bay leaf ✓ 2 medium-sized tomatoes cut into pieces ✓ ½ cup diced green bell bell pepper ✓ ½ cup diced sweet onion	✓ ¼ cup diced hot pepper ✓ ¼ cup diced celery ✓ 2 tablespoons olive oil ✓ ¾ teaspoon flavored vinegar ✓ ¼ teaspoon freshly ground black pepper

Directions:	❖ Take a large bowl and add the peanuts, diced vegetables. ❖ Whisk the olive oil, lemon juice and pepper in another bowl. ❖ Pour the mixture over the salad and toss to combine. Enjoy!
❖ Boil your peanuts for 1 minute and rinse them. ❖ The skin will be soft, so discard it. ❖ Add 2 cups of water to the Instant Pot. Add the bay leaf and the peanuts. ❖ Close the lid and cook on high pressure for 20 minutes. Drain the water.	

153) BAKED SMOKED BROCCOLI WITH GARLIC

Preparation Time:	Cooking Time:	Servings:

Ingredients:

- ✓ cooking spray
- ✓ 1 tablespoon extra-virgin olive oil
- ✓ 3 cloves garlic, minced
- ✓ 1/2 teaspoon sea salt
- ✓ 1/4 teaspoon ground black pepper

Ingredients:

- ✓ ½ teaspoon cumin
- ✓ ½ teaspoon annatto seeds
- ✓ 3 1/2 cups sliced broccoli
- ✓ 1 lime, cut into wedges
- ✓ 1 tablespoon chopped fresh cilantro

Directions:

- ❖ Preheat oven to 450 degrees F. Line a baking sheet with aluminum foil and grease with olive oil.
- ❖ Mix the olive oil, garlic, cumin, annatto seeds, salt and pepper in a bowl.

- ❖ Add the cauliflower, carrots and broccoli and combine until well coated. Spread them in a single layer on the baking sheet.
- ❖ Add the lime wedges. Roast in the oven until the vegetables caramelize, about 25 minutes.
- ❖ Remove the lime wedges and add the cilantro.

154) ROASTED CAULIFLOWER AND LIMA BEANS

Preparation Time:	Cooking Time:	Servings:

Ingredients:

- ✓ cooking spray
- ✓ 1 tablespoon melted vegan butter/margarine
- ✓ 9 garlic cloves, minced
- ✓ 1/2 teaspoon sea salt
- ✓ 1/4 teaspoon ground black pepper

Ingredients:

- ✓ 1 1/2 cups sliced cauliflower
- ✓ 3 1/2 cups cherry tomatoes
- ✓ 1 (15-ounce) can lima beans, drained
- ✓ 1 lemon, cut into wedges

Directions:

- ❖ Preheat oven to 450 degrees F. Line a baking sheet with aluminum foil and grease with melted vegan butter or margarine.
- ❖ Mix the olive oil, garlic, salt and pepper in a bowl.

- ❖ Add the cauliflower, tomatoes and lima beans. Spread them in a single layer on the baking sheet.
- ❖ Add the lemon wedges.
- ❖ Roast in the oven until the vegetables caramelize, about 25 minutes. Remove the lemon wedges.

155) THAI SPICY ROASTED BLACK BEANS AND CHOY SUM

Preparation Time:	Cooking Time:	Servings:

Ingredients:

- ✓ 1 tablespoon sesame oil
- ✓ 3 garlic cloves, minced
- ✓ 1/2 teaspoon sea salt
- ✓ 1 tablespoon Thai chili paste
- ✓ 1/4 teaspoon ground black pepper

Ingredients:

- ✓ 3 1/2 cups Choy Sum, coarsely chopped
- ✓ 2 1/2 cups cherry tomatoes
- ✓ 1 (15-ounce) can black beans, drained
- ✓ 1 lime, cut into wedges
- ✓ 1 tablespoon chopped fresh cilantro

- ❖ Preheat oven to 450 degrees F. Line a baking sheet with aluminum foil and grease it with sesame oil.
- ❖ Mix the olive oil, garlic, salt, Thai chili paste and pepper in a bowl.
- ❖ Add the choy sum, tomatoes and black beans.

- ❖ Spread them in a single layer on the baking sheet.
- ❖ Add the lime wedges. Roast in the oven until the vegetables caramelize, about 25 minutes.
- ❖ Remove the lime wedges and add the cilantro.

156) PLAIN ROASTED BROCCOLI AND CAULIFLOWER

Preparation Time:	Cooking Time:	Servings:

Ingredients:	Ingredients:
✓ 1 tablespoon extra virgin olive oil ✓ 3 cloves minced garlic ✓ 1/2 teaspoon sea salt ✓ 1/4 teaspoon ground black pepper	✓ 3 1/2 cups broccoli ✓ 2 1/2 cups cauliflower ✓ 1 tablespoon chopped fresh thyme

Directions: ❖ Preheat oven to 450 degrees F. ❖ Line a baking sheet with aluminum foil and grease with olive oil. Mix the olive oil, garlic, salt and pepper in a bowl.	❖ Add the cauliflower and tomatoes and combine until well coated. ❖ Spread them out in a single layer on the baking sheet. ❖ Roast in the oven until the vegetables caramelize, about 25 minutes. Top with the thyme. Simple

157) ROASTED NAPA CABBAGE AND EXTRA TURNIPS

Preparation Time:	Cooking Time:	Servings:

Ingredients:	Ingredients:
✓ cooking spray ✓ 1 tablespoon extra virgin olive oil ✓ 1/2 teaspoon sea salt	✓ 1/4 teaspoon ground black pepper ✓ 1/2 medium Napa cabbage, thinly sliced ✓ 1 medium turnip, thinly sliced

Directions: ❖ Preheat oven to 450 degrees F. ❖ Line a baking sheet with aluminum foil and grease with olive oil. ❖ Mix the extra ingredients together well.	❖ Add the main ingredients and combine until well coated. ❖ Spread in a single layer on the baking sheet. ❖ Roast in oven until vegetables become caramelized, about 25 minutes.

158) SIMPLE ROASTED CABBAGE WITH ARTICHOKE HEART AND EXTRA CHOY SUM

Preparation Time:	Cooking Time:	Servings:

Ingredients:	Ingredients:
✓ 1 tablespoon extra virgin olive oil ✓ 1/2 teaspoon sea salt ✓ 1/4 teaspoon ground black pepper Main ingredients	✓ 1 bunch cabbage, rinsed and drained ✓ 1 cup canned artichoke hearts ✓ 1/2 medium-flowered Chinese cabbage (choy sum), roughly chopped

Directions: ❖ Preheat oven to 450 degrees F. Line a baking sheet with aluminum foil and grease with olive oil. ❖ Mix the extra ingredients together well.	❖ Add the main ingredients and combine until well coated. ❖ Spread in a single layer on the baking sheet. ❖ Roast in oven until vegetables become caramelized, about 25 minutes.

159) ROASTED CABBAGE AND BOK CHOY EXTRA

Preparation Time:	Cooking Time:	Servings:

Ingredients:

- ✓ 1 tablespoon extra virgin olive oil
- ✓ 1/2 teaspoon sea salt
- ✓ 1/4 teaspoon ground black pepper

Directions:

- ❖ Preheat oven to 450 degrees F.
- ❖ Line a baking sheet with aluminum foil and grease with olive oil.
- ❖ Mix the extra ingredients together well.

Ingredients:

- ✓ 1 bunch kale, rinsed and drained
- ✓ 1 bunch bok choy, rinsed, drained and coarsely chopped

- ❖ Add the main ingredients and combine until well coated.
- ❖ Spread in a single layer on the baking sheet.
- ❖ Roast in oven until vegetables become caramelized, about 25 minutes.

160) ROASTED SOY BEANS AND WINTER SQUASH

Preparation Time:	Cooking Time:	Servings:

Ingredients:

- ✓ 2 (15-ounce) cans of soybeans, rinsed and drained
- ✓ 1/2 winter squash - peeled, seeded and cut into 1-inch pieces 1 red onion, diced
- ✓ 1 sweet potato, peeled and cut into 1-inch cubes
- ✓ 2 large carrots, cut into 1-inch pieces
- ✓ 3 medium potatoes
- ✓ 4 tablespoons extra virgin olive oil Ingredients for seasoning

Ingredients:

- ✓ 1 teaspoon salt
- ✓ 1/2 teaspoon ground black pepper
- ✓ 1 teaspoon onion powder
- ✓ 1 teaspoon dried basil
- ✓ 1 teaspoon Italian seasoning Ingredients for garnishes
- ✓ 2 green onions, chopped (optional)

Directions:

- ❖ Preheat oven to 350 degrees F.
- ❖ Grease baking sheet. Combine beans, squash, onion, sweet potato, carrots and russet potatoes on prepared baking sheet. Drizzle with oil and toss to coat.
- ❖ Combine the dressing ingredients in a bowl, spread over the vegetables on the baking sheet and toss to coat with the dressing.

- ❖ Bake in the oven for 25 minutes. Stir often until the vegetables are soft and lightly browned and the beans are crisp, about 20-25 minutes more.
- ❖ Season with more salt and black pepper to taste, add green onion before serving.

161) ROASTED CHAMPIGNON MUSHROOMS AND PUMPKIN

Preparation Time:	Cooking Time:	Servings:

Ingredients:

- ✓ 2 (15-ounce) cans button mushrooms, rinsed and drained
- ✓ 1/2 summer squash - peeled, seeded and cut into 1-inch pieces
- ✓ 1 red onion, diced
- ✓ 2 large turnips, cut into 1-inch pieces
- ✓ 2 large parsnips, cut into 1-inch pieces
- ✓ 3 medium potatoes, cut into 1-inch pieces
- ✓ 3 tablespoons butter Ingredients for seasoning

Ingredients:

- ✓ 1 teaspoon salt
- ✓ 1/2 teaspoon ground black pepper
- ✓ 1 teaspoon onion powder
- ✓ 2 teaspoons garlic powder
- ✓ 1 teaspoon Herbes de Provence Ingredients for garnishes
- ✓ 2 sprigs thyme, chopped (optional)

Directions:

- ❖ Preheat oven to 350 degrees F.
- ❖ Grease baking dish. Combine main ingredients on prepared baking sheet.
- ❖ Drizzle with melted butter or margarine and toss to coat. Combine the topping ingredients in a bowl, spread over the vegetables on the baking sheet and stir to coat with the toppings.

- ❖ Bake for 25 minutes. Stir often until the vegetables are soft and lightly browned and the chickpeas are crisp, about another 20-25 minutes.
- ❖ Season with more salt and black pepper to taste, add thyme before serving.

---

162) ROASTED TOMATOES RUTABAGA AND KOHLRABI

Preparation Time:	Cooking Time:	Servings:

Ingredients:

- ✓ 3 large tomatoes, cut into 1-inch pieces
- ✓ 3 red onion, diced
- ✓ 1 rutabaga, peeled and cut into 1-inch cubes
- ✓ 2 large carrots, cut into 1-inch pieces
- ✓ 3 medium kohlrabi, cut into 1-inch pieces
- ✓ 3 tablespoons extra virgin olive oil Ingredients for seasoning
- ✓ 1 teaspoon salt

Ingredients:

- ✓ 1/2 teaspoon ground black pepper
- ✓ 1 teaspoon onion powder
- ✓ 2 teaspoons garlic powder
- ✓ 1 teaspoon Spanish paprika
- ✓ 1 teaspoon cumin Ingredients for garnishes
- ✓ 2 sprigs parsley, chopped (optional)

Directions:

- ❖ Preheat oven to 350 degrees F. Grease baking sheet. Combine main ingredients on prepared baking sheet.
- ❖ Drizzle with oil and toss to coat. Combine dressing ingredients in a bowl, spread over vegetables on baking sheet and toss to coat with dressing.

- ❖ Bake in the oven for 25 minutes. Stir often until vegetables are soft, about 20-25 minutes more.
- ❖ Season with more salt and black pepper to taste, add parsley before serving.

163) BRUSSELS SPROUTS AND ROASTED BROCCOLI

Preparation Time:	Cooking Time:	Servings:

Ingredients:

- ✓ 1 large broccoli, sliced
- ✓ 1 cup bean sprouts
- ✓ 1 red onion, diced
- ✓ 3 large kohlrabi, cut into 1-inch pieces
- ✓ 2 large carrots, cut into 1-inch pieces
- ✓ 3 medium potatoes, cut into 1-inch pieces
- ✓ 3 tablespoons extra virgin olive oil Ingredients for dressing

Ingredients:

- ✓ 1 teaspoon salt
- ✓ 1/2 teaspoon ground black pepper
- ✓ 1 teaspoon onion powder
- ✓ 2 teaspoons garlic powder
- ✓ 1 teaspoon ground fennel seeds
- ✓ 1 teaspoon dried rubbed sage Ingredients for garnishes
- ✓ 2 green onions, chopped (optional)

Directions:

- ❖ Preheat oven to 350 degrees F. Grease baking sheet.
- ❖ Combine main ingredients on prepared baking sheet. Drizzle with oil and toss to coat.
- ❖ Combine dressing ingredients in a bowl, spread over vegetables on baking sheet and toss to coat with dressing. Bake in the oven for 25 minutes.

- ❖ Stir often until the vegetables are soft and lightly browned and the chickpeas are crisp, about 20-25 more minutes.
- ❖ Season with more salt and black pepper to taste, add green onion before serving.

---

164) ROASTED BROCCOLI, SWEET POTATOES AND BEAN SPROUTS

Preparation Time:	Cooking Time:	Servings:

Ingredients:

- ✓ 1 large broccoli, sliced
- ✓ 1 cup bean sprouts
- ✓ 1 yellow onion, diced
- ✓ 1 sweet potato, peeled and cut into 1-inch cubes
- ✓ 2 large carrots, cut into 1-inch pieces
- ✓ 3 medium potatoes, cut into 1-inch pieces
- ✓ 3 tablespoons canola oil Ingredients for the dressing

Ingredients:

- ✓ 1 teaspoon salt
- ✓ 1/2 teaspoon ground black pepper
- ✓ 1 teaspoon onion powder
- ✓ 2 teaspoons garlic powder
- ✓ ½ cup grated gouda cheese
- ✓ ¼ cup Parmesan cheese
- ✓ 2 green onions, chopped (optional)

Directions:

- ❖ Preheat oven to 350 degrees F. Grease baking dish. Combine main ingredients on prepared baking sheet. Drizzle with oil and toss to coat.
- ❖ Combine dressing ingredients in a bowl, spread over vegetables on baking sheet and toss to coat with dressing. Bake in the oven for 25 minutes.

- ❖ Stir often until the vegetables are soft and lightly browned and the chickpeas are crisp, about another 20-25 minutes.
- ❖ Season with more salt and black pepper to taste, add green onion before serving.

165) SWEET POTATOES AND ROASTED RED BEETS

Preparation Time:	Cooking Time:	Servings:

Ingredients:

- ✓ 1 ½ cups Brussels sprouts, cut
- ✓ 1 cup large sweet potatoes, chopped
- ✓ 1 cup large carrots, chopped
- ✓ 1 ½ cups broccoli florets

Directions:

- ❖ Preheat the oven to 425 degrees F (220 degrees C).
- ❖ Set the rack to the second lowest level of the oven. Pour lightly salted water into a bowl.
- ❖ Soak Brussels sprouts in salted water for 15 minutes and drain.

Ingredients:

- ✓ 1 cup diced red beets
- ✓ 1/2 cup yellow onion, chopped
- ✓ 2 tablespoons sesame seed oil salt and ground black pepper to taste

- ❖ Place the rest of the ingredients in a bowl.
- ❖ Spread the vegetables in a single layer on a baking sheet.
- ❖ Roast in the oven until the vegetables begin to brown and cook, about 45 minutes.

166) BEETS AND BROCCOLI FLORETS BAKED SICHUAN STYLE

Preparation Time:	Cooking Time:	Servings:

Ingredients:

- ✓ 1 ½ cups Brussels sprouts, chopped
- ✓ 1 cup broccoli florets
- ✓ 1 cup Choggia beets, chopped
- ✓ 1 ½ cups cauliflower florets

Directions:

- ❖ Preheat the oven to 425 degrees F (220 degrees C).
- ❖ Set the rack to the second lowest level of the oven. Pour lightly salted water into a bowl.

Ingredients:

- ✓ 1 cup button mushrooms, sliced
- ✓ 1/2 cup chopped red onion
- ✓ 2 tablespoons sesame oil
- ✓ ½ teaspoon Sichuan pepper salt ground black pepper to taste

- ❖ Soak Brussels sprouts in salted water for 15 minutes and drain. Place the rest of the ingredients in a bowl.
- ❖ Spread the vegetables in a single layer on a baking sheet.
- ❖ Roast in the oven until the vegetables begin to brown and cook, about 45 minutes.

167) BAKED ENOKI AND MINI CABBAGE

Preparation Time:	Cooking Time:	Servings:

Ingredients:

- ✓ 1 ½ cups mini cabbage, chopped
- ✓ 1 cup broccoli florets
- ✓ 1 cup enoki mushrooms, sliced
- ✓ 1 ½ cups cauliflower florets

Directions:

- ❖ Preheat the oven to 425 degrees F (220 degrees C).
- ❖ Set the rack to the second lowest level of the oven.
- ❖ Pour lightly salted water into a bowl. Soak Brussels sprouts in salted water for 15 minutes and drain.

Ingredients:

- ✓ 1 cup oyster mushrooms
- ✓ 1/2 cup chopped red onion
- ✓ 2 tablespoons olive oil salt and ground black pepper to taste

- ❖ Place the rest of the ingredients in a bowl.
- ❖ Spread the vegetables in a single layer on a baking sheet.
- ❖ Roast in the oven until the vegetables begin to brown and cook, about 45 minutes.

168)   TRIPLE ROASTED MUSHROOMS

Preparation Time:	Cooking Time:	Servings:

Ingredients:	Ingredients:
✓ 2 cups spinach, rinsed ✓ 1 cup oyster mushrooms ✓ 1 cup button mushrooms, sliced ✓ 1 ½ cups enoki mushrooms	✓ 1/2 cup chopped red onion ✓ 2 tablespoons extra virgin olive oil salt and ground black pepper to taste ✓ 1/4 cup ricotta cheese

Directions:

❖ Preheat the oven to 425 degrees F (220 degrees C).

❖ Set the rack to the second lowest level of the oven. Pour lightly salted water into a bowl.

❖ Soak spinach in salted water for 15 minutes and drain.

❖ Place the rest of the ingredients in a bowl.

❖ Spread the vegetables in a single layer on a baking sheet. Roast in the oven until the vegetables begin to brown and cook, about 45 minutes.

169)   MINI ROASTED CABBAGE AND SWEET POTATOES

Preparation Time:	Cooking Time:	Servings:

Ingredients:	Ingredients:
✓ 1 ½ cups mini cabbage, cut ✓ 1 cup large pieces of potatoes ✓ 1 cup large pieces of rainbow carrots ✓ 1 ½ cup pieces of potatoes	✓ 1 cup parsnips ✓ 1/2 cup pieces of red onion ✓ 2 tablespoons extra virgin olive oil Sea salt Rainbow pepper to taste ✓ 1/4 cup cottage cheese

Directions:

❖ Preheat the oven to 425 degrees F (220 degrees C).

❖ Set the rack to the second lowest level of the oven. Pour lightly salted water into a bowl.

❖ Soak mini cabbage in salted water for 15 minutes and drain.

❖ Place the rest of the ingredients in a bowl. Spread the vegetables in a single layer on a baking sheet.

❖ Roast in the oven until the vegetables begin to brown and cook, about 45 minutes.

Chapter 3. DINNER

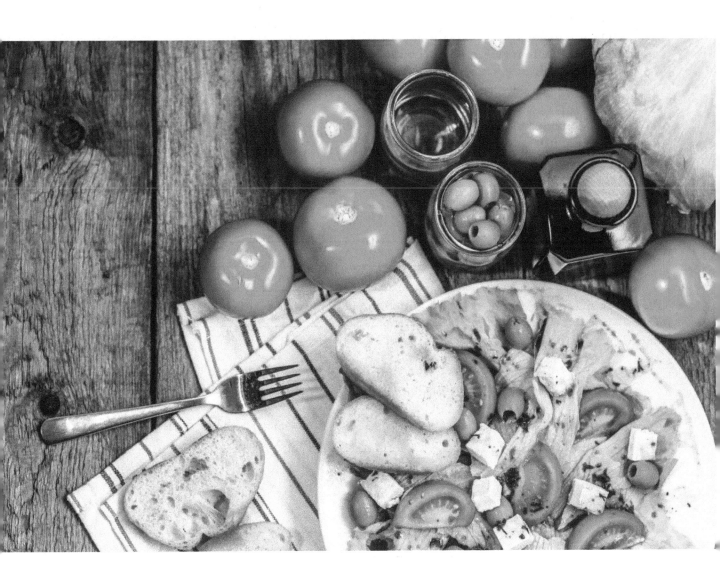

170) CURRIED BEEF MEATBALLS

Preparation Time: 20 minutes	**Cooking Time:** 22 minutes	**Servings: 6**

Ingredients:

- ✓ For the meatballs:
- ✓ 1 pound lean ground beef
- ✓ 2 organic eggs, bea10
- ✓ 3 tablespoons red onion, chopped
- ✓ ¼ cup fresh basil leaves, chopped
- ✓ 1 (1-inch) piece fresh ginger, finely chopped
- ✓ 4 cloves garlic, finely chopped
- ✓ 3 Thai bird's eye chilies, chopped
- ✓ 1 tablespoon coconut sugar
- ✓ 1 tablespoon red curry paste - Salt, to taste –
- ✓ 1 tablespoon fish sauce

Ingredients:

- ✓ 2 tablespoons coconut oil

  For Curry:
- ✓ 1 red onion, chopped - Salt, to taste
- ✓ 4 garlic cloves, chopped
- ✓ 1 piece fresh ginger (1 inch), chopped
- ✓ 2 Thai chilies, chopped
- ✓ 2 tablespoons red curry paste
- ✓ 1 coconut milk (14 ounces) - Salt and freshly ground black pepper, to taste
- ✓ Lime wedge, to serve

Directions:

- ❖ For meatballs in a large bowl, add all ingredients except oil and mix until well combined. Make small balls from the mixture. In a large skillet, melt the coconut oil over medium heat. Add the patties and cook for about 3-5 minutes or until golden brown on all sides.

- ❖ Transfer the meatballs to a bowl. In the same skillet, add the onion and a pinch of salt and sauté for about 5 minutes. Add the garlic, ginger and chilies and sauté for about 1 minute. Add the curry paste and stir-fry for about 1 minute.
- ❖ Add the coconut milk and meatballs and bring to a boil over low heat. Reduce heat to low and simmer, covered for about 10 minutes. Serve with the lime wedge dressing.

171) GRILLED STEAK WITH COCONUT

Preparation Time: 15 minutes	**Cooking Time:** 8-9 minutes	**Servings: 4**

Ingredients:

- ✓ 2 teaspoons fresh ginger, finely grated
- ✓ 2 teaspoons fresh lime zest, finely grated
- ✓ ¼ cup coconut sugar
- ✓ 2 teaspoons fish sauce

Ingredients:

- ✓ 2 tablespoons fresh lime juice
- ✓ ½ cup coconut milk
- ✓ 1 pound beef skirt steak, trimmed and cut into 4-inch slices lengthwise
- ✓ Salt, to taste

Directions:

- ❖ In a resealable bag, mix all ingredients except steak and salt. Add the steak and coat generously with the marinade. Seal the bag and refrigerate to marinate for about 4-12 hours. Preheat grill to high heat. Grease the grill grate. Remove the steak from the refrigerator and discard the marinade.

- ❖ Using a paper towel, pat the steak dry and sprinkle with salt evenly. Cook the steak for about 3 1/2 minutes. Turn the middle side out and cook for about 2½ to 5 minutes or until desired doneness.
- ❖ Remove from grill pan and hold side for about 5 minutes before slicing. Using a clear, crisp knife, cut into desired slices and serve.

	172) **LAMB WITH PRUNES**	
Preparation Time: 15 minutes	**Cooking Time:** a couple of hours and 40 minutes	**Servings: 4-6**

Ingredients:

- ✓ 3 tablespoons coconut oil
- ✓ 2 onions, finely chopped
- ✓ 1 (1-inch) piece of fresh ginger, chopped
- ✓ 3 garlic cloves, chopped
- ✓ ½ teaspoon turmeric powder
- ✓ 2 ½ lbs. of lamb shoulder, trimmed and cut into 3-inch cubes

Ingredients:

- ✓ Salt and freshly ground black pepper, to taste
- ✓ ½ teaspoon saffron threads, crumbled
- ✓ 1 cinnamon stick
- ✓ 3 cups water
- ✓ 1 cup runes, pitted and halved

Directions:

- ❖ In a large skillet, melt the coconut oil over medium heat. Add the onions, ginger, garlic cloves and turmeric and sauté for about 3-5 minutes. Sprinkle the lamb evenly with salt and black pepper. In the skillet, add the lamb and saffron threads and cook for about 4-5 minutes.

- ❖ Add the cinnamon stick and water and produce to a boil over high heat. Reduce the heat to low and simmer, covered for about 1½-120 minutes or until the lamb has reached the desired temperature.
- ❖ Add the plums and simmer for about 20½ hours. Remove the cinnamon stick and serve hot.

	173) **GROUND LAMB WITH PEAS**	
Preparation Time: 15 minutes	**Cooking Time:** 55 minutes	**Servings: 4**

Ingredients:

- ✓ 1 tablespoon coconut oil
- ✓ 3 dried red chilies
- ✓ 1 cinnamon stick (2 inches)
- ✓ 3 green cardamom pods
- ✓ ½ teaspoon cumin seeds
- ✓ 1 medium red onion, chopped
- ✓ 1 piece fresh ginger (¾ inch), chopped
- ✓ 4 cloves garlic, minced
- ✓ 1½ teaspoons ground coriander
- ✓ ½ teaspoon garam masala
- ✓ ½ teaspoon ground cumin

Ingredients:

- ✓ ½ teaspoon ground turmeric
- ✓ ¼ teaspoon ground nutmeg
- ✓ 2 bay leaves
- ✓ 1 pound ground lean lamb
- ✓ ½ cup Roma tomatoes, chopped
- ✓ 1-1½ cup water
- ✓ 1 cup fresh green peas, shelled
- ✓ 2 tablespoons plain Greek yogurt, whipped
- ✓ ¼ cup fresh cilantro, chopped
- ✓ Salt and freshly ground black pepper, to taste

Directions:

- ❖ In a Dutch oven, melt the coconut oil over medium-high heat. Add the red chiles, cinnamon stick, cardamom pods and cumin seeds and sauté for about thirty seconds. Add the onion and sauté for about 3-4 minutes.

- ❖ Add the ginger, garlic cloves and spices and sauté for about thirty seconds. Add the lamb and cook about 5 minutes. Add the tomatoes and cook about 10 minutes. Add the water and green peas and cook covered for about 25-30 minutes.
- ❖ Add the yogurt, cilantro, salt and black pepper and cook for about 4-5 minutes. Serve hot.

174) ROAST LAMB CHOPS

Preparation Time: 15 minutes	**Cooking Time:** half an hour	**Servings: 4**

Ingredients:

For the lamb marinade:
- ✓ 4 cloves garlic, chopped
- ✓ 1 (2 inch) piece fresh ginger, chopped
- ✓ 2 green chiles, seeded and chopped
- ✓ 1 teaspoon fresh lime zest
- ✓ 2 teaspoons garam masala
- ✓ 1 teaspoon ground coriander
- ✓ 1 teaspoon ground cumin
- ✓ ½ teaspoon ground cinnamon
- ✓ 1 teaspoon coconut oil, melted
- ✓ 2 tablespoons fresh lime juice
- ✓ 6-7 tablespoons plain Greek yogurt
- ✓ 1 (8-bone) rack of lamb, chopped

Ingredients:
- ✓ 2 onions, sliced

For Relish:
- ✓ ½ of garlic, chopped
- ✓ 1 (1-inch) piece of fresh ginger, chopped
- ✓ ¼ cup fresh cilantro, chopped
- ✓ ¼ cup fresh mint, chopped
- ✓ 1 green chile, seeded and chopped
- ✓ 1 teaspoon fresh lime zest
- ✓ 1 teaspoon organic honey
- ✓ 2 tablespoons fresh apple juice
- ✓ 2 tablespoons fresh lime juice

❖ For the chops in a very mixer, add all ingredients except the yogurt, chops and onions and pulse until smooth. Transfer the mixture to a large bowl with the yogurt and stir to combine well. Add the chops and coat generously with the mixture. Refrigerate to marinate for about twenty-four hours.

❖ Preheat oven to 375 degrees F. Line baking sheet with aluminum foil. Place the onion wedges in the bottom of the prepared baking dish. Arrange rack of lamb on top of onion wedges. Roast about half an hour. Meanwhile for relish in blender, add all ingredients and pulse until smooth. Serve the chops and onions along with the relish.

175) MEATBALLS BAKED WITH SHALLOTS

Preparation Time: 20 minutes	**Cooking Time:** 35 minutes	**Servings: 4-6**

Ingredients:

For the patties:
- ✓ 1 lemongrass stalk, outer peel peeled and chopped
- ✓ 1 (1½-inch) piece fresh ginger, sliced –
- ✓ 3 garlic cloves, chopped
- ✓ 1 cup fresh cilantro leaves, coarsely chopped
- ✓ ½ cup fresh basil leaves, coarsely chopped
- ✓ 2 tablespoons plus 1 teaspoon fish sauce
- ✓ 2 tablespoons water
- ✓ 2 tablespoons fresh lime juice

Ingredients:
- ✓ ½ pound lean ground pork
- ✓ 1 pound lean ground lamb
- ✓ 1 carrot, peeled and grated
- ✓ 1 organic egg, bea10
- ✓ For the scallions: -
- ✓ 16 scallion stalks, chopped
- ✓ 2 tablespoons coconut oil, melted - Salt, to taste
- ✓ ½ cup water

Directions:

❖ Preheat oven to 375 degrees F. Grease a baking sheet. In a blender, add the lemongrass, ginger, garlic, fresh herbs, fish sauce, water and lime juice and blend until finely chopped.

❖ Transfer the amalgam to a bowl with the remaining ingredients and mix until well combined. Make 1-inch balls from the mixture.

❖ Arrange the balls in the prepared baking dish in a single layer. In another rimmed baking dish, arrange shallot stalks in a single layer. Drizzle with coconut oil and sprinkle with salt. Pour the water into the baking dish and cover 1 tightly with aluminum foil.

❖ Cook the shallots for about half an hour.. Bake the meatballs for about 30-35 minutes. Pork with peppers This stir-fry doesn't just taste wonderful, it's also full of nutritious benefits.

176)	PORK CHILI	
Preparation Time: 15 minutes	**Cooking Time**: 60 minutes	**Servings**: 8

Ingredients:

- ✓ 2 tbsp. organic extra virgin olive oil
- ✓ 2 lbs. ground pork
- ✓ 1 medium red bell pepper, seeded and chopped
- ✓ 1 medium onion, chopped
- ✓ 5 cloves of garlic, finely chopped
- ✓ 1 part (2 in.) of chili pepper, ground
- ✓ 1 tablespoon ground cumin
- ✓ 1 teaspoon ground turmeric

Ingredients:

- ✓ 3 tablespoons chili powder
- ✓ ½ teaspoon chipotle chili powder - Salt and freshly ground black pepper, to taste
- ✓ 1 cup chicken broth
- ✓ 1 (28-ounce) can fire-roasted tomatoes, crushed
- ✓ 2 medium bokchoy heads, sliced
- ✓ 1 avocado, peeled, pitted and chopped

Directions:

- ❖ In a large skillet, heat oil over medium heat. Add the pork and sauté for about 5 minutes. Add the bell bell pepper, onion, garlic, chili and spices and sauté for about 5 minutes. Add the broth and tomatoes and bring to a boil.
- ❖

- ❖ Add the bokchoy and cook, covered for about twenty minutes. Uncover and cook for about 20 ½ hours. Serve warm while using an avocado garnish.

177)	PORK MEATBALLS AND BAKED MUSHROOMS	
Preparation Time: 15 minutes	**Cooking Time**: 15 minutes	**Servings**: 6

Ingredients:

- ✓ 1 pound lean pork
- ✓ 1 egg white,
- ✓ 4 fresh shiitake mushrooms, cut and chopped
- ✓ 1 tablespoon fresh parsley, chopped
- ✓ 1 tablespoon fresh basil leaves, chopped

Ingredients:

- ✓ 1 tablespoon fresh mint leaves, chopped
- ✓ 2 teaspoons fresh lemon zest, finely grated
- ✓ 1½ teaspoons fresh ginger, finely grated
- ✓ Salt and freshly ground black pepper, to taste

Directions:

- ❖ Preheat the oven to 425 degrees F. Place the rack in the center of the oven. Line a baking sheet with parchment paper. In a sizable bowl, add all ingredients and mix until well combined.

- ❖ Make small balls of equal size from the mixture. Arrange the balls on the prepared baking sheet in a single layer. Bake for about 12 quarters of an hour or until cooked through.

178) BEEF WITH CITRUS FRUITS AND BOK CHOY

Preparation Time: 15 minutes	**Cooking Time**: 11 minutes	**Servings**: 4

Ingredients:

For the marinade:
- ✓ 2 cloves minced garlic
- ✓ 1 (1-inch) piece fresh ginger, grated
- ✓ 1/3 cup fresh orange juice
- ✓ ½ cup coconut aminos
- ✓ 2 teaspoons fish sauce
- ✓ 2 teaspoons Sriracha
- ✓ 1¼ pounds sirloin steak, thinly sliced and cut

Ingredients:

For the vegetables:
- ✓ 2 tablespoons coconut oil, divided
- ✓ 3-4 wide strips of fresh orange zest
- ✓ 1 jalapeño bell pepper, thinly sliced
- ✓ ½ pound green beans, cut and halved crosswise
- ✓ 1 tablespoon arrowroot powder
- ✓ ½ pound bokchoy, chopped
- ✓ 2 teaspoons sesame seeds

Directions:

❖ For the marinade in a large bowl, mix together garlic, ginger, orange juice, coconut aminos, fish sauce and Sriracha. Add beef and coat generously with marinade. Refrigerate to marinate for about a couple of hours. In a substantial skillet, heat oil over medium-high heat. Add the orange zest and sauté about 2 minutes.

❖ Remove the beef from the bowl, reserving the marinade. In the skillet, add the beef and increase the heat to high.

❖ Sauté for about 2-3 minutes or until golden brown. Using a slotted spoon, transfer the beef and orange strips to a bowl. Using a paper towel, pat the pan dry. In a similar skillet, heat the remaining oil over medium-high heat.

❖ Add the jalapeño bell pepper and green beans and sauté for about 3-4 minutes. Meanwhile, add the arrowroot powder to the reserved marinade and stir to combine. In the skillet, add the marinade mixture, beef and bokchoy and cook for about 1-2 minutes. Serve hot with sesame seed garnish.

179) GROUND BEEF WITH CABBAGE

Preparation Time: 10 minutes	**Cooking Time**: 15 minutes	**Servings**: 6

Ingredients:

- ✓ 1 tablespoon olive oil
- ✓ 1 onion, thinly sliced
- ✓ 2 teaspoons fresh ginger, chopped
- ✓ 4 cloves garlic, chopped
- ✓ 1 pound lean ground beef

Ingredients:

- ✓ 1½ tablespoons fish sauce
- ✓ 2 tablespoons fresh lime juice
- ✓ 1 small head of purple cabbage, shredded
- ✓ 2 tablespoons peanut butter
- ✓ ½ cup fresh cilantro, chopped

Directions:

❖ In a large skillet, heat the oil over medium heat. Add the onion, ginger and garlic and sauté for about 4-5 minutes. Add the beef and cook for about 7-8 minutes, breaking it up with a spoon.

❖ Drain off the extra liquid in the skillet. Stir in the fish sauce and lime juice and cook for about 1 minute. Add the cabbage and cook about 4-5 minutes or until desired doneness. Add the peanut butter and cilantro and cook for about 1 minute. Serve hot.

180) BEEF CHILI WITH VEGETABLES

Preparation Time: 15 minutes	**Cooking Time**: 1 hour	**Servings**: 6-8

Ingredients:

- ✓ 2 lbs. lean ground beef
- ✓ - ½ head of cauliflower, cut into large pieces
- ✓ - 1 onion, chopped
- ✓ - 6 cloves of garlic, chopped
- ✓ - 2 cups of pumpkin puree
- ✓ - 1 tsp. dried oregano, crushed
- ✓ - 1 tsp. dried thyme, crushed
- ✓ - 1 teaspoon ground cumin
- ✓ - 1 teaspoon ground turmeric

Ingredients:

- ✓ - 1-2 teaspoons chili powder
- ✓ - 1 teaspoon paprika
- ✓ - 1 teaspoon cayenne pepper
- ✓ - ¼ teaspoon red pepper flakes, crushed - Salt and freshly ground black pepper, to taste
- ✓ - 1 (26-ounce) can tomatoes, drained
- ✓ - ½ cup water
- ✓ - 1 cup meat stock

Directions:

❖ Heat a substantial skillet over medium-high heat. Add the beef and sauté for about 5 minutes. Add the cauliflower, onion and garlic and sauté for about 5 minutes.

❖ Add the spices and herbs and stir to mix well. Reduce heat to low and simmer, covered for about 30-45 minutes. Serve hot.

181) BEEF MEATBALLS IN TOMATO SAUCE

Preparation Time: 20 minutes	**Cooking Time**: 37 minutes	**Servings**: 4

Ingredients:

For the meatballs:
- ✓ - 1 pound lean ground beef
- ✓ - 1 organic egg
- ✓ - 1 tablespoon fresh ginger, chopped
- ✓ - 1 garlic oil, chopped
- ✓ - 2 tablespoons fresh cilantro, finely chopped
- ✓ - 2 tablespoons tomato paste
- ✓ - 1/3 cup almond flour
- ✓ - 1 tablespoon ground cumin –
- ✓ Pinch of ground cinnamon - Salt and freshly ground black pepper, to taste
- ✓ - ¼ cup coconut oil

Ingredients:

For the tomato sauce:
- ✓ - 2 tablespoons coconut oil
- ✓ - ½ small onion, chopped
- ✓ - 2 cloves garlic, chopped
- ✓ - 1 teaspoon fresh lemon zest, finely grated
- ✓ - 2 cups tomatoes, finely chopped
- ✓ - Pinch of ground cinnamon
- ✓ - 1 teaspoon red pepper flakes, crushed
- ✓ - ¾ cup chicken broth - Salt and freshly ground black pepper, to taste
- ✓ - ¼ cup fresh parsley, chopped

Directions:

❖ For the meatballs, in a large bowl, add all ingredients except oil and mix until well combined. Make balls about 1 inch from the mixture. In a substantial skillet, melt the coconut oil over medium heat. Add the patties and cook for about 3-5 minutes or until golden brown on all sides.

❖ Transfer the meatballs to a bowl. For the sauce in a large skillet, melt the coconut oil over medium heat. Add the onion and garlic and sauté about 4 minutes. Add the lemon zest and sauté about 1 minute.

❖ Add the tomatoes, cinnamon, red pepper flakes and broth and simmer about 7 minutes. Add the salt, black pepper and meatballs and reduce the heat to medium-low. Simmer for about twenty minutes. Serve hot with all the parsley garnishes.

182) SPICY LAMB CURRY

Preparation Time: 15 minutes	**Cooking Time**: 2 quarter hours	**Servings**: 6-8

Ingredients:

For the spice blend:
- ✓ - 4 teaspoons ground coriander
- ✓ - 4 teaspoons ground cumin
- ✓ - ¾ teaspoon ground ginger
- ✓ - 2 teaspoons ground cinnamon
- ✓ - ½ teaspoon ground cloves
- ✓ - ½ teaspoon ground cardamom
- ✓ - 2 tablespoons sweet paprika
- ✓ - ½ teaspoon cayenne pepper
- ✓ - 2 teaspoons chili powder

Ingredients:

- ✓ - 2 teaspoons salt

For the Curry:
- ✓ - 1 tablespoon coconut oil
- ✓ - 2 pounds boneless lamb, trimmed and cut into 1-inch cubes - Salt and freshly ground black pepper, to taste
- ✓ - 2 cups onions, chopped
- ✓ - 1¼ cups water
- ✓ - 1 cup coconut milk

Directions:

❖ For the spice mixture in a bowl, mix together all the spices. Keep aside. Season lamb with salt and black pepper. In a large Dutch oven, heat oil over medium-high heat. Add the lamb and sauté for about 5 minutes.

❖ Add the onion and cook about 4-5 minutes. Add the spice mixture and cook for about 1 minute. Add the water and coconut milk and bring to a boil over high heat. Reduce heat to low and simmer, covered for about 1-120 minutes or until desired doneness of lamb. Uncover and simmer for about 3-4 minutes. Serve hot.

---

183) GROUND LAMB WITH HARISSA

Preparation Time: 15 minutes	**Cooking Time**: 1 hour 11 minutes	**Servings**: 4

Ingredients:

- ✓ 1 tablespoon extra virgin olive oil
- ✓ - 2 red peppers, seeded and finely chopped
- ✓ - 1 yellow onion, finely chopped
- ✓ - 2 cloves of garlic, finely chopped
- ✓ - 1 teaspoon ground cumin
- ✓ - ½ teaspoon ground turmeric

Ingredients:

- ✓ - ¼ teaspoon ground cinnamon
- ✓ - ¼ teaspoon ground ginger
- ✓ - 1 1/2 pounds ground lean lamb - Salt, to taste
- ✓ - 1 can diced tomatoes
- ✓ - 2 tablespoons harissa
- ✓ - 1 cup water - Fresh chopped cilantro, for garnish

Directions:

❖ In a large skillet, heat the oil over medium-high heat. Add the bell bell pepper, onion and garlic and sauté for about 5 minutes. Add the spices and sauté for about 1 minute. Add the lamb and salt and cook about 5 minutes, breaking it up into pieces.

❖ Add the tomatoes, harissa and water and bring to a boil. Reduce the heat to low and simmer, covered for about 1 hour. Serve hot while using the harissa garnish.

184) PAN-FRIED LAMB CHOPS

Preparation Time: 10 minutes	**Cooking Time**: 4-6 minutes	**Servings: 4**

Ingredients:

- ✓ 4 cloves of garlic, peeled - Salt, to taste
- ✓ - 1 teaspoon black mustard seeds, finely crushed
- ✓ - 2 teaspoons ground cumin
- ✓ - 1 teaspoon ground ginger

Ingredients:

- ✓ - 1 teaspoon ground coriander
- ✓ - ½ teaspoon ground cinnamon - Fresh ground black pepper, to taste.
- ✓ - 1 tablespoon coconut oil
- ✓ - 8 medium lamb chops, sliced

Directions:

❖ Place the garlic cloves on a cutting board and sprinkle with a little salt. Using a knife, crush the garlic until it forms a paste. In a bowl, mix together the garlic paste and spices.

❖ With a clear, crisp knife, make 3-4 cuts on both sides in the chops. Generously rub the chops with the garlic mixture. In a large skillet, melt the butter over medium heat. Add chops and cook for about 2-3 minutes per side or until desired doneness.

185) LAMB AND PINEAPPLE KEBAB

Preparation Time: 15 minutes	**Cooking Time**: 10 minutes	**Servings: 4-6**

Ingredients:

- ✓ 1 large pineapple, cut into 1½-inch cubes, split
- ✓ - 1 piece fresh ginger (½ inch), chopped
- ✓ - 2 cloves garlic, chopped - Salt, to taste

Ingredients:

- ✓
- ✓ - 16- to 24-ounce lamb shoulder steak, cut and diced into 1½-inch cubes –
- ✓ Fresh mint leaves from a bunch
- ✓ - Cinnamon powder, to taste

Directions:

❖ In a blender, add about 1 1/2 servings of pineapple, the ginger, garlic, and salt, and blend until smooth. Transfer the amalgam to a large bowl. Add chops and coat generously with mixture.

❖ Refrigerate to marinate for about 1-2 hours. Preheat grill to medium heat. Grease the grill grate. Thread lam, remaining pineapple, and mint leaves onto pre-soaked wooden skewers. Grill skewers for about 10 minutes, turning occasionally.

	186)	SPICED PORK ONE	

Preparation Time: 15 minutes	**Cooking Time:** 60 minutes	**Servings: 6**

Ingredients:

- ✓ 1 (2-inch) piece of fresh ginger, chopped
- ✓ - 5-10 cloves of garlic, chopped
- ✓ - 1 teaspoon ground cumin
- ✓ - ½ teaspoon ground turmeric
- ✓ 1 tablespoon ground hot paprika
- ✓ - 1 tablespoon red pepper flakes - Salt, to taste
- ✓ - 2 tablespoons cider vinegar
- ✓ - 2 pounds pork shoulder, chopped and diced
- ✓ 1½ inches

Ingredients:

- ✓ - 2 cups domestic hot water, divided
- ✓ - 1 (1 inch wide) ball of tamarind pulp
- ✓ - ¼ cup olive oil
- ✓ - 1 teaspoon black mustard seeds, crushed
- ✓ - 4 green cardamoms
- ✓ - 5 whole cloves
- ✓ - 1 (3 inch) cinnamon stick
- ✓ - 1 cup onion, finely chopped
- ✓ - 1 large red bell pepper, seeded and chopped

Directions:

❖ In a food processor, add the ginger, garlic, cumin, turmeric, paprika, red pepper flakes, salt, and apple cider vinegar and pulse until smooth. Transfer the amalgam to a large bowl. Add the pork and coat generously with the mixture.

❖ Set aside, covered for about an hour at room temperature. In a bowl, add 1 cup hot water and tamarind and set aside until water cools. Using your hands, mash the tamarind to extract the pulp .

❖ Add the remaining cup of hot water and stir until well combined. Through a fine sieve, strain the tamarind juice into a bowl. In a large skillet, heat the oil over medium-high heat. Add the mustard seeds, green cardamoms, cloves and cinnamon stick and sauté for about 4 minutes.

❖ Add the onion and sauté for about 5 minutes. Add the pork and sauté for about 6 minutes. Add the tamarind juice and bring to a boil. Reduce heat to medium-low and simmer for 1 1/2 hours. Stir in bell bell pepper and cook for about 7 minutes.

	187)	PORK CHOPS IN CREAMY SAUCE	

Preparation Time: 15 minutes	**Cooking Time:** 14 minutes	**Servings: 4**

Ingredients:

- ✓ 2 garlic cloves, chopped
- ✓ - 1 small jalapeño bell pepper, chopped
- ✓ - ¼ cup fresh cilantro leaves
- ✓ - 1½ teaspoons turmeric powder, divided
- ✓ - 1 tablespoon fish sauce
- ✓ - 2 tablespoons fresh lime juice

Ingredients:

- ✓ - 1 can coconut milk (13½-ounce)
- ✓ - 4 pork chops (½-inch thick)
- ✓ - Salt, to taste
- ✓ - 1 tablespoon coconut oil
- ✓ - 1 shallot, finely chopped

Directions:

❖ In a blender, add the garlic, jalapeño bell pepper, cilantro, 1 teaspoon ground turmeric, fish sauce, lime juice, and coconut milk, and blend until smooth.

❖ Sprinkle the pork evenly with the salt and remaining turmeric. In a skillet, melt the butter over medium-high heat. Add the shallots and sauté about 1 minute. Add the chops and cook for about 2 minutes per side. Transfer chops to a bowl. Add the coconut mixture and bring to a boil.

❖ Reduce heat to medium and simmer, stirring occasionally for about 5 minutes. Stir in the pork chops and cook for about 3-4 minutes. Serve hot.

188) DECENT BEEF AND ONION STEW

Preparation Time: 10 minutes	**Cooking Time**: 1-2 hours	**Servings: 4**

Ingredients:

- ✓ 2 pounds lean beef, cubed
- ✓ 3 pounds shallots, peeled
- ✓ 5 garlic cloves, peeled, whole
- ✓ 3 tablespoons tomato paste

Ingredients:

- ✓ 1 bay leaf
- ✓ ¼ cup olive oil
- ✓ 3 tablespoons lemon juice

Directions:

❖ Take a stew pot and place it over medium heat. Add the olive oil and let it heat up. Add the meat and let it brown.

❖ Add the remaining ingredients and cover with water. Bring everything to a boil. Reduce the heat to low and cover the pot. Simmer for 1-2 hours until meat is cooked through. Serve hot!

189) BEEF SAUTEED WITH ZUCCHINI AND CILANTRO

Preparation Time: 10 minutes	**Cooking Time**: 10 minutes	**Servings: 4**

Ingredients:

- ✓ 10 ounces beef, cut into 1-2-inch strips
- ✓ 1 zucchini, cut into 2-inch strips
- ✓ ¼ cup parsley, chopped

Ingredients:

- ✓ 3 cloves garlic, chopped
- ✓ 2 tablespoons tamari sauce
- ✓ 4 tablespoons avocado oil

Directions:

❖ Add 2 tablespoons avocado oil to a skillet over high heat. Place the beef strips in and sauté for a few minutes over high heat.

❖ Once the meat is brown, add the zucchini strips and sauté until tender. Once tender, add the tamari sauce, garlic, parsley and let them sit for a few more minutes. Serve immediately and enjoy!

190) WALNUT AND ASPARAGUS DELIGHT

Preparation Time: 5 minutes	**Cooking Time**: 5 minutes	**Servings: 4**

Ingredients:

- ✓ 1 ½ tablespoons olive oil
- ✓ ¾ pound asparagus, chopped

Ingredients:

- ✓ ¼ cup walnuts, chopped Sunflower seeds and pepper to taste

Directions:

❖ Place a skillet over medium heat, add the olive oil and let it heat up. Add asparagus and saute for 5 minutes until browned.

❖ Season with sunflower seeds and pepper. Remove from heat. Add walnuts and toss to combine. Serve hot!

191) BEEF SOUP

Preparation Time: 10 minutes	**Cooking Time:** 40 minutes	**Servings: 4**

Ingredients:

- ✓ 1 pound ground beef, lean
- ✓ 1 cup mixed vegetables, frozen
- ✓ 1 yellow onion, chopped

Ingredients:

- ✓ 6 cups vegetable broth
- ✓ 1 cup low-fat cream
- ✓ Pepper to taste

Directions:

❖ Take a pot and add all ingredients except heavy cream, salt and black pepper. Bring to a boil. Reduce heat to a simmer.

❖ Cook for 40 minutes. Once cooked, heat the heavy cream. Then add once the soup is cooked. Blend the soup until smooth using an immersion blender. Season with salt and black pepper. Serve and enjoy!

192) CLEANED CHICKEN AND MUSHROOM STEW

Preparation Time: 10 minutes	**Cooking Time:** 35 minutes	**Servings: 4**

Ingredients:

- ✓ 4 chicken breast halves, cut into bite-sized pieces
- ✓ 1 pound mushrooms, sliced (5-6 cups)
- ✓ 1 bunch onion, chopped

Ingredients:

- ✓ 4 tablespoons olive oil
- ✓ 1 teaspoon thyme Sunflower seeds and pepper as needed

Directions:

❖ Take a large deep skillet and place it over medium-high heat. Add the oil and let it heat up. Add the chicken and cook for 4-5 minutes per side until lightly browned.

❖ Add the spring onions and mushrooms, season with the sunflower seeds and pepper to your taste. Stir. Cover with the lid and bring the mixture to a boil. Reduce heat and simmer for 25 minutes. Serve.

193) ZUCCHINI ZOODLES WITH CHICKEN AND BASIL

Preparation Time: 10 minutes	**Cooking Time:** 10 minutes	**Servings: 2**

Ingredients:

- ✓ 2 chicken fillets, diced
- ✓ 2 tablespoons ghee
- ✓ 1 pound tomatoes, diced
- ✓ ½ cup basil, chopped

Ingredients:

- ✓ ¼ cup coconut milk
- ✓ 1 garlic clove, peeled, chopped
- ✓ 1 zucchini, chopped

Directions:

❖ Fry the diced chicken in the ghee until no longer pink. Add the tomatoes and season with the sunflower seeds. Simmer and reduce the liquid. Prepare your Zucchini Zoodles by chopping the zucchini in a food processor.

❖ Add the basil, garlic, coconut milk and almonds to the chicken and cook for a few minutes. Add half of the Zucchini Zoodles to a bowl and top with the creamy tomato basil chicken. Enjoy!

194) THE GOODNESS OF BREADED CHICKEN WITH ALMONDS

Preparation Time: 15 minutes	Cooking Time: 15 minutes	Servings: 3

Ingredients:

- ✓ 2 large chicken breasts, boneless and skinless
- ✓ 1/3 cup lemon juice
- ✓ 1 ½ cups seasoned almond flour

Ingredients:

- ✓ 2 tablespoons coconut oil Lemon pepper, to taste
- ✓ Parsley for garnish

Directions:

- ❖ Cut the chicken breast in half. Pound each half until ¼ inch thick. Take a skillet and place it over medium heat, add the oil and heat it up. Dip each slice of chicken breast into the lemon juice and let it sit for 2 minutes.

- ❖ Flip and let the other side rest for 2 minutes. Transfer to almond flour and coat both sides. Add the coated chicken to the oil and fry for 4 minutes per side, making sure to liberally sprinkle the lemon pepper.
- ❖ Transfer to a paper-lined sheet and repeat until all chicken is fried. Garnish with parsley and enjoy!

195) PORK CHOPS WITH ALMOND BUTTER

Preparation Time: 5 minutes	Cooking Time: 25 minutes	Servings: 2

Ingredients:

- ✓ 1 tablespoon almond butter, divided
- ✓ 2 boneless pork chops Pepper to taste

Ingredients:

- ✓ 1 tablespoon dry, low-fat, low-sodium Italian seasoning
- ✓ 1 tablespoon olive oil

Directions:

- ❖ preheat oven to 350 degrees F. Pat pork chops dry with a paper towel and place in a baking dish. Season with pepper and Italian seasoning.

- ❖ Drizzle pork chops with olive oil. Top each chop with ½ tablespoon almond butter. Bake for 25 minutes. Transfer pork chops to two plates and top with almond butter. Serve and enjoy!

196) HEALTHY MEDITERRANEAN LAMB CHOPS

Preparation Time: 10 minutes	Cooking Time: 10 minutes	Servings: 4

Ingredients:

- ✓ 4 lamb shoulder chops,
- ✓ 8 ounces each
- ✓ 2 tablespoons Dijon mustard

Ingredients:

- ✓ 2 tablespoons balsamic vinegar
- ✓ ½ cup olive oil
- ✓ 2 tablespoons chopped fresh basil

Directions:

- ❖ Dry the lamb chops with a kitchen towel and place them on a shallow glass baking dish. Take a bowl and whisk in Dijon mustard, balsamic vinegar, and pepper and mix well.
- ❖ Very slowly whisk the oil into the marinade until the mixture is smooth Stir in the basil. Pour the marinade over the lamb chops and stir to coat both sides well. Cover the ribs and let them marinate for 1-4 hours (in a cool place).

- ❖ Remove the ribs and let them sit for 30 minutes to allow the temperature to reach a normal level. Preheat grill to medium heat and add oil to grill.
- ❖ Grill the lamb chops for 5-10 minutes per side until both sides are golden brown. When the center reads 145 degrees F, the ribs are ready, serve and enjoy!

197) DUCK BREAST WITH BROWN BUTTER

Preparation Time: 5 minutes	Cooking Time: 25 minutes	Servings: 3

Ingredients:

- ✓ 1 whole
- ✓ 6-ounce duck breast, with skin Pepper to taste
- ✓ 1 head of radicchio, 4 ounces, coreless

Ingredients:

- ✓ ¼ cup unsalted butter
- ✓ 6 fresh sage leaves, sliced

Directions:

- ❖ Preheat oven to 400 degrees F. Dry duck breast with paper towel. Season with the pepper. Place the duck breast in a skillet and place over medium heat, sear for 3-4 minutes each side. Turn the breast and transfer the pan to the oven. Roast for 10 minutes (uncovered).

- ❖ Cut the radicchio in half. Remove and discard the woody white core and thinly slice the leaves. Keep them aside. Remove the pan from the oven. Transfer the duck breast, fat side up, to the cutting board and let it rest.
- ❖ Reheat the skillet over medium heat. Add the unsalted butter and sage and cook for 3-4 minutes. Cut the duck into 6 equal slices. Divide the radicchio between 2 plates, top with the duck breast slices and drizzle with browned butter and sage. Enjoy!

198) CAULIFLOWER BREAD STICK

Preparation Time: 10 minutes	Cooking Time: 48 minutes	Servings: 5

Ingredients:

- ✓ 1 cup cashew/ricotta kite cheese
- ✓ 1 tablespoon organic almond butter
- ✓ 1 whole egg
- ✓ ½ teaspoon Italian seasoning
- ✓ ¼ teaspoon red pepper flakes

Ingredients:

- ✓ 1/8 teaspoon kosher sunflower seeds
- ✓ 2 cups cauliflower rice, cooked for 3 minutes in the microwave
- ✓ 3 teaspoons garlic, minced
- ✓ Parmesan, grated

Directions:

- ❖ Preheat oven to 350 degrees F. Add almond butter to a small skillet and melt over low heat Add red pepper flakes, garlic to almond butter and cook for 2-3 minutes. Add the garlic and almond butter mixture to the bowl with the cooked cauliflower and add the Italian seasoning. Season with the sunflower seeds and toss, refrigerate for 10 minutes.

- ❖ Add the cheese and eggs to the bowl and mix. Place a layer of parchment paper in the bottom of a 9 x 9 baking dish and grease with cooking spray, add the egg and mozzarella mixture to the cauliflower mixture.
- ❖ Add the mixture to the baking dish and smooth it out to a thin layer with the palms of your hand. Bake for 30 minutes, remove from oven and top with a few shakes of parmesan and mozzarella cheese. Bake for an additional 8 minutes. Enjoy!

199) CHICKEN WITH CHIPOTLE LETTUCE

Preparation Time: 10 minutes	Cooking Time: 25 minutes	Servings: 6

Ingredients:

- ✓ 1 pound chicken breast, cut into strips
- ✓ Drizzle with olive oil
- ✓ 1 red onion, finely sliced
- ✓ 14 ounces tomatoes
- ✓ 1 teaspoon chipotle, chopped

Ingredients:

- ✓ ½ teaspoon cumin
- ✓ Lettuce as needed
- ✓ Fresh cilantro leaves
- ✓ Jalapeno chiles, sliced
- ✓ Fresh tomato slices for garnish Lime wedge

- ❖ Take a non-stick skillet and place it over medium heat. Add the oil and heat it up. Add the chicken and cook until it turns brown. Keep the chicken aside. Add the tomatoes, sugar, chipotle, and cumin to the same pan and simmer for 25 minutes until you have a nice sauce.

- ❖ Add the chicken to the sauce and cook for 5 minutes. Transfer the mixture to another place. Use lettuce strips to take a portion of the mixture and serve with a squeeze of lemon. Enjoy!

200) CREAMED CORN DISH

Preparation Time: 10 minutes	**Cooking Time**: 4 hour	**Servings: 3**

Ingredients:

- ✓ 3 cups corn
- ✓ 2 ounces cream cheese, cubed
- ✓ 2 tablespoons milk
- ✓ 2 tablespoons whipping cream

Ingredients:

- ✓ 2 tablespoons melted butter
- ✓ Salt and pepper to taste
- ✓ 1 tablespoon green onion, chopped

Directions:

- ❖ Add the corn, cream cheese, milk, whipping cream, butter, salt and pepper to your Slow Cooker. Give it a good stir to mix everything well.

- ❖ Put the lid on and cook on LOW for 4 hours. Divide the mixture between serving plates. Serve and enjoy!

201) ETHIOPIAN CABBAGE DELIGHT

Preparation Time: 15 minutes	**Cooking Time**: 6-8 hour	**Servings: 6**

Ingredients:

- ✓ ½ cup water
- ✓ 1 head of kale, chopped and shredded
- ✓ 1 pound sweet potatoes, peeled and shredded
- ✓ 3 carrots, peeled and shredded
- ✓ 1 onion, sliced

Ingredients:

- ✓ 1 teaspoon extra virgin olive oil
- ✓ ½ teaspoon turmeric powder
- ✓ ½ teaspoon cumin powder
- ✓ ¼ teaspoon ginger powder

Directions:

- ❖ Add water to your Slow Cooker. Take a medium bowl and add cabbage, carrots, sweet potatoes, onion and mix.

- ❖ Add the olive oil, turmeric, ginger, cumin and stir until the vegetables are completely coated. Transfer the vegetable mix to your Slow Cooker.
- ❖ Cover and cook on LOW for 6-8 hours. Serve and enjoy!

202) FRESH HARMONY OF APPLES AND CARROTS

Preparation Time: 10 minutes	**Cooking Time**: 10 minutes	**Servings: 6**

Ingredients:

- ✓ 1 cup apple juice
- ✓ 1 pound baby carrots

Ingredients:

- ✓ 1 tablespoon cornstarch
- ✓ 1 tablespoon chopped mint

Directions:

- ❖ Add the apple juice, carrots, cornstarch and mint to your Instant Pot. Stir and close the lid.

- ❖ Cook on high pressure for 10 minutes. Perform a quick release. Divide the mix among plates and serve. Enjoy!

203) BLACK PEAS AND SPINACH DISH

Preparation Time: 10 minutes	**Cooking Time:** 8 hours	**Servings: 4**

Ingredients:

- ✓ 1 cup black peas, soaked overnight and drained
- ✓ 2 cups low-sodium vegetable broth
- ✓ 1 can (15 ounces) tomatoes, diced with juice
- ✓ 8 ounces ham, chopped
- ✓ 1 onion, chopped
- ✓ 2 cloves garlic, chopped

Ingredients:

- ✓ 1 teaspoon dried oregano
- ✓ 1 teaspoon salt
- ✓ ½ teaspoon freshly ground black pepper
- ✓ ½ teaspoon ground mustard
- ✓ 1 bay leaf

Directions:

- ❖ Add the ingredients listed in your Slow Cooker and stir. Put the lid on and cook on LOW for 8 hours. Discard the bay leaf. Serve and enjoy!

204) CABBAGE AND APPLES IN SWEET AND SOUR SAUCE

Preparation Time: 15 minutes	**Cooking Time:** 8 hours	**Servings: 4**

Ingredients:

- ✓ ¼ cup honey
- ✓ ¼ cup apple cider vinegar
- ✓ 2 tablespoons orange-garlic sauce
- ✓ 1 teaspoon sea salt

Ingredients:

- ✓ 3 tart sweet apples, peeled, pitted and sliced
- ✓ 2 heads of collard greens, pitted and chopped
- ✓ 1 sweet red onion, thinly sliced

Directions:

- ❖ Take a small bowl and whisk together the honey, orange garlic and chili sauce, and vinegar. Mix well. Add the honey mixture, apples, onion and cabbage to your Slow Cooker and stir.

- ❖ Close the lid and cook on LOW for 8 hours. Serve and enjoy!

205) GARLIC SAUCE WITH ORANGE AND CHILI PEPPER

Preparation Time: 15 minutes	**Cooking Time:** 8 hours	**Servings: 5**

Ingredients:

- ✓ ½ cup apple cider vinegar
- ✓ 4 pounds red jalapeno peppers, stems, seeds and ribs removed, chopped
- ✓ 10 cloves garlic, chopped
- ✓ ½ cup tomato paste

Ingredients:

- ✓ Juice of 1 orange peel
- ✓ ½ cup honey
- ✓ 2 tablespoons soy sauce
- ✓ 2 teaspoons salt

- ❖ Add the vinegar, garlic, peppers, tomato paste, orange juice, honey, zest, soy sauce and salt to your Slow Cooker. Stir and close the lid. Cook on LOW for 8 hours. Use as needed

206) VEGETABLE BROTH FOR EVERY DAY

Preparation Time: 5 minutes	**Cooking Time**: 8-12 hours	**Servings: 10**

Ingredients:

- ✓ 2 celery stalks (with leaves), quartered
- ✓ 4 ounces mushrooms, with stalks
- ✓ 2 carrots, unpeeled and quartered
- ✓ 1 onion, unpeeled, quartered pole to pole
- ✓ 1 garlic head, unpeeled, halved in center

Ingredients:

- ✓ 2 sprigs fresh thyme
- ✓ 10 peppercorns
- ✓ ½ teaspoon salt
- ✓ Enough water to fill 3 quarts of Slow Cooker

Directions:

- ❖ Add celery, mushrooms, onion, carrots, garlic, thyme, salt, pepper and water to pot over low heat. Stir and cover.

- ❖ Cook on LOW for 8-12 hours. Strain broth through a fine mesh cloth/wire mesh and discard solids. Use as needed.

207) CARAMELIZED PORK CHOPS AND ONION

Preparation Time: 5 minutes	**Cooking Time**: 40 minutes	**Servings: 4**

Ingredients:

- ✓ Roast 4-pound beef
- ✓ 4 ounces green chile, minced
- ✓ 2 tablespoons chili powder

Ingredients:

- ✓ ½ teaspoon dried oregano
- ✓ ½ teaspoon cumin, ground
- ✓ 2 cloves garlic, minced

Directions:

- ❖ Rub the chops with a seasoning of 1 teaspoon pepper and 2 teaspoons sunflower seeds. Take a skillet and place it over medium heat, add the oil and let the oil heat up Brown the seasoned chops on both sides.

- ❖ Add the water and onion to the skillet and cover, lower the heat to low and simmer for 20 minutes. Turn the chops over and season with more sunflower seeds and pepper. Cover and cook until the water evaporates completely and the beer shows a slightly brown consistency.
- ❖ Remove chops and serve with a caramelized onion garnish. Serve and enjoy!

208) APPLE PIE CRACKERS

Preparation Time: 10 minutes	**Cooking Time**: 2 hours	**Servings: 100 crackers**

Ingredients:

- ✓ 2 tablespoons + 2 teaspoons avocado oil
- ✓ 1 medium Granny Smith apple, coarsely chopped
- ✓ ¼ cup erythritol
- ✓ 1/4 cup sunflower seeds, coarsely ground
- ✓ 1 ¾ cup flax seeds, coarsely ground

Ingredients:

- ✓ 1/8 teaspoon clove powder
- ✓ 1/8 teaspoon cardamom powder
- ✓ 3 tablespoons nutmeg
- ✓ ¼ teaspoon ginger powder

Directions:

- ❖ Preheat oven to 225 degrees F. Line two baking sheets with baking paper and set aside. Add the oil, apple, and erythritol to a bowl and mix.

- ❖ Transfer to a food processor and add remaining ingredients, process until combined. Transfer batter to baking sheets, spread evenly and cut into crackers. Bake for 1 hour, turn and bake for another hour. Let them cool and serve. Enjoy!

209)   GROUND BEEF AND VEGETABLE CURRY

Preparation Time: 15 minutes	**Cooking Time**: 36 minutes	**Servings**: 6-8

Ingredients:

- ✓ 2-3 tablespoons coconut oil
- ✓ - 1 cup onion, chopped
- ✓ - 1 clove garlic, chopped
- ✓ - 1 pound lean ground beef –
- ✓   1½ tablespoons curry powder
- ✓ - 1/8 teaspoon ginger powder

Ingredients:

- ✓ - 1/8 teaspoon cinnamon powder
- ✓ - 1/8 teaspoon turmeric powder
- ✓ - Salt, to taste
- ✓ - 2½-3 cups tomatoes, finely chopped
- ✓ - 2½-3 cups fresh peas, shelled
- ✓ - 2 sweet potatoes, peeled and chopped

Directions:

- ❖ In a large skillet, melt the coconut oil over medium heat. Add the onion and garlic and sauté for about 4-5 minutes. Add the beef and cook for about 4-5 minutes.

- ❖ Add the curry powder and spices and cook for about 1 minute. Add the tomatoes, peas and sweet potato and bring to a boil over low heat. Simmer, covered for about 25 minutes.

210)   HONEY GLAZED BEEF

Preparation Time: quarter hour	**Cooking Time**: 12 minutes	**Servings**: 2-3

Ingredients:

- ✓ 2 Tablespoons arrowroot flour - Salt and freshly ground black pepper, to taste
- ✓ - 1 lb. beefsteak, cut into ¼ inch thick slices
- ✓ - ½ cup plus 1 tbsp. coconut oil, divided –
- ✓   2 cloves minced garlic
- ✓ - 1 teaspoon ground ginger

Ingredients:

- ✓ - Pinch of red pepper flakes, crushed
- ✓ - 1/3 cup organic honey
- ✓ - ½ cup beef broth
- ✓ - ½ cup coconut aminos
- ✓   - 3 shallots, chopped

Directions:

- ❖ In a bowl, mix together the arrowroot flour, salt and black pepper. Coat the beef slices in the arrowroot flour mixture evenly after which get rid of the excess mixture. Set aside for about 10-15 minutes. For the sauce in a skillet, melt 1 tablespoon of coconut oil over medium heat.
- ❖ Add the garlic, ginger powder and red pepper flakes and sauté for about 1 minute. Add the honey, broth and coconut amino acid and stir to mix well. Increase the heat to high and cook, stirring constantly for about 3 minutes. Remove from heat and set aside. In a large skillet, melt the remaining coconut oil over medium heat. Add beef and stir-fry about 2-3 minutes.

- ❖ Transfer beef to a paper towel-lined plate to drain. Remove the oil from the pan and return the beef to the pan. Sauté for about 1 minute. Add the honey sauce and cook for about 3 minutes. Add the shallot and cook for about 1 minute. Serve hot.

211) ROAST LAMB WITH SPINACH

Preparation Time: quarter hour	**Cooking Time:** 55 minutes	**Servings: 6**

Ingredients:

- ✓ 2 tablespoons coconut oil
- ✓ - 2 pounds lamb necks, trimmed and cut into 2-inch pieces crosswise
- ✓ - Salt, to taste
- ✓ - 2 medium onions, chopped
- ✓ - 3 tablespoons fresh ginger, chopped
- ✓ - 4 cloves garlic, chopped
- ✓ - 2 tablespoons ground coriander
- ✓ - 1 tablespoon ground cumin
- ✓ - 1 teaspoon ground turmeric

Ingredients:

- ✓ - ¼ cup coconut milk
- ✓ - ½ cup tomatoes, chopped
- ✓ - 2 cups boiling water
- ✓ - 30 ounces frozen spinach, thawed and squeezed
- ✓ - 1½ tablespoons garam masala
- ✓ - 1 tablespoon fresh lemon juice
- ✓ - Freshly ground black pepper, to taste

Directions:

❖ Preheat oven to 300 degrees F. In a substantial Dutch oven, melt the coconut oil over medium-high heat. Add the lamb necks and sprinkle with salt. Sauté about 4-5 minutes or until completely browned.

❖ Transfer the lamb to a plate and lower the heat to medium. In the same pan, add the onion and sauté for about 10 minutes. Add the ginger, garlic and spices and sauté for about 1 minute.

❖ Add the coconut milk and tomatoes and cook about 3-4 minutes. Using an immersion blender, blend the mixture until smooth. Add the lamb, boiling water and salt and bring to a boil. Cover the pot and transfer to the oven.

❖ Bake about 2 1/2 hours. Now, remove the pan from the oven and place on medium heat. Stir in the spinach and garam masala and cook for about 3-5 minutes. Add the fresh lemon juice, salt and black pepper and remove from heat. Serve hot.

212) GRILLED SHOULDER OF LAMB

Preparation Time: 10 minutes	**Cooking Time:** 8-10 minutes	**Servings: 10**

Ingredients:

- ✓ 2 tablespoons fresh ginger, chopped
- ✓ - 2 tablespoons garlic, chopped
- ✓ - ¼ cup fresh lemongrass, chopped
- ✓ - ¼ cup fresh orange juice

Ingredients:

- ✓ - ¼ cup coconut aminos
- ✓ - freshly ground black pepper, to taste
- ✓ - 2 pounds lamb shoulder, chopped

Directions:

❖ In a bowl, mix all ingredients except lamb shoulder. In a baking dish, mash the lamb shoulder and generously coat the lamb with half of the marinade mixture. Reserve the remaining mixture. Refrigerate to marinate overnight.

❖ Preheat the broiler in the oven. Place a rack inside a broiler pan and arrange about 4-5 inches from the heating unit. Remove lamb shoulder from refrigerator and remove excess marinade. Bake for about 4-5 minutes on both sides. Serve with all the reserved marinade as a sauce.

213)   LAMB BURGERS WITH AVOCADO SAUCE

Preparation Time: 20 minutes	**Cooking Time**: 10 minutes	**Servings**: 4-6

Ingredients:

For the burgers:
- ✓ - 1 (2 inch) piece of fresh ginger, grated
- ✓ - 1 pound of lean ground lamb
- ✓ - 1 medium onion, grated
- ✓ - 2 cloves of garlic, minced
- ✓ - 1 bunch of fresh mint leaves, finely chopped
- ✓ - 2 teaspoons ground coriander
- ✓ - 2 teaspoons ground cumin
- ✓ - ½ teaspoon ground allspice
- ✓ - ½ teaspoon ground cinnamon
- - Salt and freshly ground black pepper, to taste
- ✓ - 1 tablespoon essential olive oil

Ingredients:

For the sauce:
- ✓ - 3 small cucumbers, peeled and grated
- ✓ - 1 avocado, peeled, pitted and chopped
- ✓ - ½ of garlic oil, crushed
- ✓ - 2 tablespoons fresh lemon juice
- ✓ - 2 tablespoons olive oil
- ✓ - 2 tablespoons fresh dill, finely chopped
- ✓ - 2 tablespoons chives, finely chopped
- ✓ - Salt and freshly ground black pepper, to taste

Directions:

❖ Preheat oven rack. Lightly grease a broiler pan. For burgers in a large bowl, squeeze ginger juice. Add the remaining ingredients and mix until well combined. Make equal-sized burgers from your mixture.

❖ Place the burgers in a broiler pan and cook about 5 minutes per side. Meanwhile for the dip squeeze the juice from the cucumbers into a bowl. In a blender, add the avocado, garlic, lemon juice and oil and blend until smooth.

❖ Transfer the avocado mixture to a bowl. Add the remaining ingredients and stir to mix. Serve the burgers with the avocado sauce.

214)   PORK WITH PINEAPPLE

Preparation Time: 15 minutes	**Cooking Time**: 14 minutes	**Servings**: 4

Ingredients:

- ✓ 2 tablespoons coconut oil
- ✓ - 1½ pound pork
- ✓ 10 derloin, trimmed and cut into bite-size pieces
- ✓ - 1 onion, chopped
- ✓ - 2 cloves garlic, chopped
- ✓ - 1 (1-inch) piece fresh ginger, chopped

Ingredients:

- ✓ - 20-ounce pineapple, chopped
- ✓ - 1 large red bell bell pepper, seeded and chopped
- ✓ - ¼ cup fresh pineapple juice
- ✓ - ¼ cup coconut aminos
- ✓ - Salt and freshly ground black pepper, to taste

Directions:

❖ In a substantial skillet, melt the coconut oil over high heat. Add pork and sauté about 4-5 minutes. Transfer pork to a bowl. In the exact same pan, heat the remaining oil over medium heat.

❖ Add the onion, garlic and ginger and sauté for about 2 minutes. Add the pineapple and bell bell pepper and sauté for about 3 minutes.

❖ Add the pork, pineapple juice and coconut amino acid and cook for about 3-4 minutes. Serve hot.

215) PORK CHOPS GLAZED WITH PEACH

Preparation Time: quarter hour	**Cooking Time:** 16 minutes	**Servings: 2**

Ingredients:

- ✓ 2 boneless pork chops
- ✓ - Salt and freshly ground black pepper, to taste
- ✓ - 1 ripe yellow peach, peeled, pitted, chopped and split
- ✓ - 1 tablespoon organic olive oil
- ✓ - 2 tablespoons shallots, chopped
- ✓ - 2 tablespoons garlic, minced

Ingredients:

- ✓ - 2 tablespoons fresh ginger, minced
- ✓ - 1 tablespoon organic honey –
- ✓ 1 tablespoon balsamic vinegar
- ✓ - 1 tablespoon coconut aminos
- ✓ - ¼ tablespoon red pepper flakes, crushed
- ✓ - ¼ cup water

Directions:

❖ Sprinkle pork chops generously with salt and black pepper. In a blender, add 1/2 of the peach and pulse until it forms a puree. Reserve the remaining peach. In a skillet, heat oil over medium heat.

❖ Add the shallots and sauté about 1-2 minutes. Add the garlic and ginger and sauté about 1 minute. Add the remaining ingredients and lower the heat to medium-low. Bring to a boil and simmer about 4-5 minutes or until a sticky glaze forms. Remove from heat and reserve 1/3 with the glaze and keep aside. Coat the chops with the remaining glaze. Heat a nonstick skillet over medium-high heat.

❖ Add the chops and sear for about 4 minutes on both sides. Transfer chops to a plate and coat with all remaining glaze evenly. Top with reserved chopped peaches and serve.

216) BEEF WITH CARROTS AND BROCCOLI

Preparation Time: 15 minutes	**Cooking Time:** 14 minutes	**Servings: 4**

Ingredients:

- ✓ 2 tablespoons coconut oil, divided
- ✓ - 2 medium garlic cloves, minced
- ✓ - 1 pound sirloin steak, trimmed and cut into thin strips
- ✓ - Salt, to taste
- ✓ - ¼ cup chicken broth
- ✓ - 2 teaspoons fresh ginger, grated

Ingredients:

- ✓ - 1 tablespoon ground flaxseed
- ✓ - ½ teaspoon red pepper flakes, crushed
- ✓ - ¼ teaspoon freshly ground black pepper –
- ✓ 1 large carrot, peeled and thinly sliced
- ✓ - 2 cups broccoli florets
- ✓ - 1 medium shallot, thinly sliced

Directions:

❖ In a substantial skillet, heat 1 tablespoon oil over medium-high heat. Add garlic and sauté about 1 minute. Add the beef and salt and cook for about 4-5 minutes or until golden brown.

❖ Using a slotted spoon, transfer the beef to a bowl. Remove the liquid from the pan. In a bowl, mix together broth, ginger, flaxseed, red pepper flakes and black pepper. In a similar skillet, heat the remaining oil over medium heat.

❖ Add carrot, broccoli and ginger mixture and cook for about 3-4 minutes or until desired doneness. Add beef and shallots and cook for about 3-4 minutes.

Chapter 4. DESSERTS

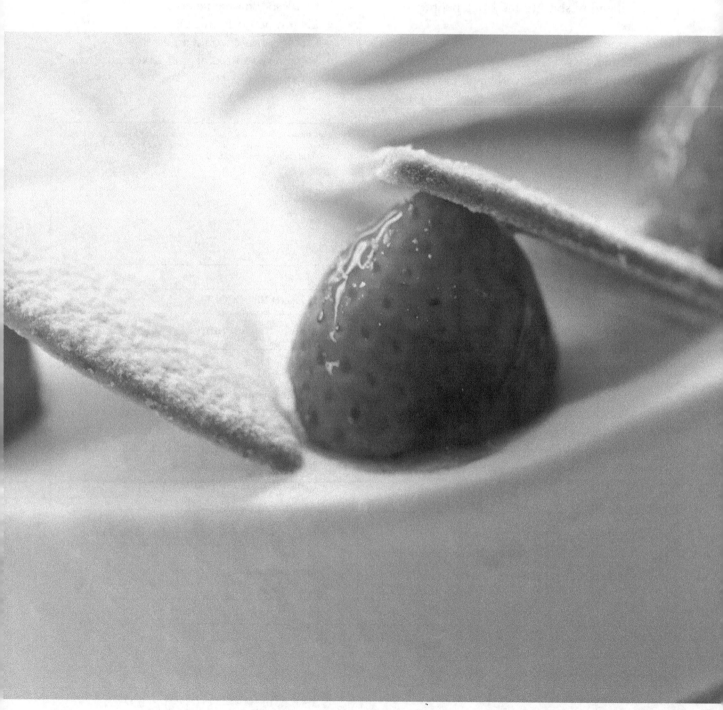

217) STRAWBERRY AND AVOCADO MEDLEY

Preparation Time:	Cooking time: 5 minutes	Servings: 4

Ingredients:	Ingredients:
✓ 2 cups strawberries, cut in half ✓ 1 avocado, pitted and sliced	✓ 2 tablespoons slivered almonds

Directions:

❖ Place all ingredients in a mixing bowl. Stir to combine. Allow to cool in the refrigerator before serving.

218) HONEY AND BERRIES GRANITA

Preparation Time: 10 minutes + freezing time	Cooking Time:	Servings: 4

Ingredients:	Ingredients:
✓ 1 teaspoon lemon juice ✓ ¼ cup honey ✓ 1 cup fresh strawberries	✓ 1 cup fresh raspberries ✓ 1 cup fresh blueberries

Directions:

❖ Bring 1 cup of water to a boil in a saucepan over high heat. Stir in honey until dissolved. Remove from heat and stir in berries and lemon juice; allow to cool.

❖ Once cooled, add mixture to a food processor and pulse until smooth. Transfer to a shallow glass and freeze for 1 hour. Stir with a fork and freeze for another 30 minutes. Repeat a couple of times. Serve in dessert dishes.

219) CHOCOLATE COVERED STRAWBERRIES

Preparation Time: 15 minutes + cooling time	Cooking Time:	Servings: 4

Ingredients:	Ingredients:
✓ 1 cup chocolate chips ✓ ¼ cup coconut flakes ✓ 1 pound strawberries	✓ ½ teaspoon vanilla extract ✓ ½ teaspoon nutmeg powder ✓ ¼ teaspoon salt

Directions:

❖ Melt chocolate chips for 30 seconds. Remove and stir in vanilla, nutmeg and salt. Allow to cool for 2-3 minutes. Dip strawberries into chocolate and then into coconut chips.

❖ Place on a cookie sheet lined with wax paper and let sit for 30 minutes until the chocolate dries. Serve.

220)	SUMMER FRUIT SORBET	

Preparation Time: 10 minutes + freezing time	**Cooking Time**:	**Servings**: 4

Ingredients:

- ✓ ¼ cup honey
- ✓ 4 cups watermelon cubes

Directions:

- ❖ In a food processor, blend the watermelon, honey and lemon juice to form a chunky puree. Transfer to a freezer-proof container and place in the freezer for 1 hour.

Ingredients:

- ✓ ¼ cup lemon juice
- ✓ 12 mint leaves to serve

- ❖ Remove container and scrape with a fork. Place back in the freezer and repeat the process every half hour until the sorbet is completely frozen, about 4 hours. Distribute into bowls, garnish with mint leaves and serve.

221)	HONEY PUDDING WITH KIWI	

Preparation Time:	**Cooking Time**:	**Servings**:

Ingredients:

- ✓ 2 kiwis, halved and sliced
- ✓ 1 egg
- ✓ 2 ¼ cups milk

Directions:

- ❖ In a bowl, beat egg with honey. Stir in 2 cups of milk and vanilla. Pour into a saucepan over medium heat and bring to a boil. Combine cornstarch and remaining milk in a bowl.

Ingredients:

- ✓ 2 kiwis, halved and sliced
- ✓ 1 egg
- ✓ 2 ¼ cups milk

- ❖ Pour slowly into the pot and boil for 1 minute until thickened, stirring often. Divide among 4 cups and transfer to refrigerator. Add the kiwis and serve.

222)	PEACH CAKE WITH WALNUTS AND RAISINS	

Preparation Time: 50 minutes + cooling time	**Cooking Time**:	**Servings**: 6

Ingredients:

- ✓ 2 peaches, peeled and chopped
- ✓ ½ cup raisins, soaked
- ✓ 1 cup regular flour
- ✓ 3 eggs
- ✓ 1 tablespoon dark rum
- ✓ ¼ teaspoon cinnamon powder
- ✓ 1 teaspoon vanilla extract
- ✓ 1 ½ teaspoons baking powder

Directions:

- ❖ Preheat oven to 350°F. In a bowl, mix the flour, cardamom cinnamon, vanilla, baking powder and salt. In another bowl, beat the eggs with the Greek yogurt using an electric mixer. Gently add the coconut and olive oil. Combine well.

Ingredients:

- ✓ 4 tablespoons Greek yogurt
- ✓ ¼ cup coconut oil
- ✓ ¼ cup olive oil
- ✓ 2 tablespoons honey
- ✓ 1 cup brown sugar
- ✓ 4 tablespoons walnuts, chopped
- ✓ ¼ teaspoon caramel sauce

- ❖ Toss in the rum, honey and sugar; stir to combine. Mix the wet ingredients with the dry mixture. Stir in the peaches, raisins and nuts. Pour the mixture into a greased baking dish and bake for 30-40 minutes until a knife inserted into the center of the cake comes out clean.
- ❖ Remove from oven and let rest for 10 minutes, then flip onto a wire rack to cool completely. Heat the caramel sauce in a skillet and pour over the cooled cake to serve.

223) HEARTY CHIA AND BLACKBERRY PUDDING

Preparation Time: 45 minutes	Cooking Time:	Servings: 2

Ingredients:

- ✓ ¼ cup chia seeds
- ✓ ½ cup blackberries, fresh
- ✓ 1 teaspoon liquid sweetener 1

Ingredients:

- ✓ cup coconut and almond milk, whole and unsweetened
- ✓ 1 teaspoon vanilla extract

Directions:

- ❖ Take the vanilla, liquid sweetener and coconut almond milk and add to the blender. Process until thick. Add the blackberries and process until smooth.

- ❖ Divide the mixture between cups and chill for 30 minutes. Serve and enjoy!

224) DELICATE BLACKBERRY CRUMBLE

Preparation Time: 10 minutes	Cooking Time: 45 minutes	Servings: 4

Ingredients:

- ✓ ½ cup coconut flour
- ✓ ½ cup banana, peeled and mashed
- ✓ 6 tablespoons water
- ✓ 3 cups fresh blackberries

Ingredients:

- ✓ ½ cup arrowroot flour
- ✓ 1 ½ teaspoons baking soda
- ✓ 4 tablespoons almond butter, melted
- ✓ 1 tablespoon fresh lemon juice

Directions:

- ❖ Preheat oven to 300 degrees F. Take a baking sheet and lightly grease it. Take a bowl and mix all ingredients except blackberries, mix well.

- ❖ Place the blackberries in the bottom of the baking dish and cover with flour. Bake for 40 minutes. Serve and enjoy!

225) AMAZING MAPLE PECAN BACON SLICES

Preparation Time: 10 minutes	Cooking Time: 25 minutes + freezing time	Servings: 12

Ingredients:

- ✓ 1 tablespoon sugar-free maple syrup
- ✓ 12 slices of bacon
- ✓ Granular Stevia to taste
- ✓ 15-20 drops of Stevia

Ingredients:

- ✓ For the coating:
- ✓ 4 tablespoons dark cocoa powder
- ✓ ¼ cup pecans, chopped
- ✓ 15-20 drops of Stevia

Directions:

- ❖ Take a baking sheet and lay the bacon slices on it. Rub with maple syrup and Stevia, turn the slices over and do the same with the other side. Bake for 10-15 minutes at 220 degrees F. After baking, drain bacon grease.

- ❖ To form a batter, mix the bacon fat, Stevia and cocoa powder. Dip the bacon slices in the batter and roll in the chopped pecans. Allow to air dry until the chocolate hardens.

226) CARROT BALL DELIGHT

Preparation Time: 10minutes	**Cooking Time**:	**Servings**: 4

Ingredients:

- ✓ 6 pitted Medjool dates
- ✓ 1 carrot, finely grated
- ✓ ¼ cup raw walnuts

Ingredients:

- ✓ ¼ cup unsweetened coconut, shredded
- ✓ 1 teaspoon nutmeg
- ✓ 1/8 teaspoon sunflower seeds

Directions:

❖ Take a food processor and add dates, ¼ cup grated carrots, coconut sunflower seeds, nutmeg. Blend well and reduce the mixture to a puree.

❖ Add the nuts and the remaining ¼ cup of carrots. Pulse the mixture until chunky in consistency. Form balls with your hand and roll them in the coconut. Top with the carrots and chill. Enjoy!

227) SPICE FRIENDLY MUFFINS

Preparation Time: 5 minutes	**Cooking Time**: 45 minutes	**Servings**: 12

Ingredients:

- ✓ ½ cup raw hemp hearts
- ✓ ½ cup flax seeds
- ✓ ¼ cup chia seeds
- ✓ 2 tablespoons Psyllium husk powder

Ingredients:

- ✓ 1 tablespoon cinnamon stevia flavor
- ✓ ½ teaspoon baking powder
- ✓ ½ teaspoon sunflower seeds
- ✓ 1 cup water

Directions:

❖ preheat oven to 350 degrees F. Line muffin tray with liners. Take a large bowl and add the peanut almond butter, pumpkin, sweetener, coconut almond milk, flax seeds and mix well. Continue to mix until the mixture has been completely combined. Take another bowl and add the baking powder, spices, and coconut flour. Mix well.

❖ Add the dry ingredients to the wet bowl and mix until the coconut flour has mixed well. Let sit for a while until the coconut flour has absorbed all the moisture.

❖ Divide the mixture between your muffin pans and bake for 45 minutes. Enjoy!

228) FANTASTIC CAULIFLOWER BAGELS

Preparation Time: 10 minutes	**Cooking Time**: 30 minutes	**Servings**: 12

Ingredients:

- ✓ 1 large cauliflower, floreted and coarsely chopped
- ✓ ¼ cup nutritional yeast
- ✓ ¼ cup almond flour
- ✓ ½ teaspoon garlic powder

Ingredients:

- ✓ 1 ½ teaspoons fine sea sunflower seeds
- ✓ 1 whole egg
- ✓ 1 tablespoon sesame seeds

❖ preheat oven to 400 degrees F. Line a baking sheet with parchment paper; set aside. Blend the cauliflower in the food processor and transfer to a bowl.

❖ Add the nutritional yeast, almond flour, garlic powder and sunflower seeds to a bowl, mix. Take another bowl and beat the eggs, add to the cauliflower mix. Give the mixture a stir. Incorporate the dough into the egg mixture.

❖ Make balls with the dough, poking a hole in each ball with your thumb. Place them on the prepared sheet, flattening them into a bagel shape. Sprinkle with sesame seeds and bake for 30 minutes. Remove from oven and let them cool, enjoy!

229) SAVORY LIME PIE

Preparation Time: 5 minutes	Cooking Time: 5 minutes + freezing time	Servings: 12

Ingredients:

- ✓ 1 tablespoon ground cinnamon
- ✓ 3 tablespoons almond butter
- ✓ 1 cup almond flour

For the filling:
- ✓ 3 tablespoons grass-fed almond butter

Ingredients:

- ✓ 4 ounces whole cream cheese
- ✓ ¼ cup coconut oil
- ✓ 2 limes
- ✓ A handful of baby spinach Stevia to taste

Directions:

❖ Mix the cinnamon and almond butter to form a crumble mixture. Press this mixture into the bottom of 12 muffin cups. Bake for 7 minutes at 350 degrees F.

❖ Squeeze the lime and grate the zest while the crust is baking. Take a food processor and add all the filling ingredients. Blend until smooth. Let cool naturally. Pour the mixture into the center. Freeze until set and serve.

230) THE PERFECT PONZU ORANGE

Preparation Time: 30 minutes	Cooking Time: 5 minutes	Servings: 8

Ingredients:

- ✓ ¼ cup coconut amino acids
- ✓ ½ cup rice vinegar
- ✓ 2 tablespoons dried fish flakes

Ingredients:

- ✓ 1 (1 inch) square kombu (kelp)
- ✓ 1 orange, quartered

Directions:

❖ Take a saucepan and place it over medium heat. Add the coconut amino acid, rice vinegar, fish flakes, kombu, and orange quarters and let the mixture sit for 30 minutes.

❖ Bring the mixture to a boil and immediately remove from heat. Allow to cool and strain through cheesecloth. Serve and enjoy!

231) THE REFRESHING NUTTER

Preparation Time: 10 minutes	Cooking Time:	Servings: 1

Ingredients:

- ✓ 1 tablespoon chia seeds
- ✓ 2 cups water 1 ounce macadamia nuts

Ingredients:

- ✓ 1-2 packets Stevia, optional
- ✓ 1 ounce hazelnuts

Directions:

❖ Add all of the listed ingredients to a blender. Blend on high speed until smooth and creamy. Enjoy your smoothie.

232) APPLE AND ALMOND MUFFINS

Preparation Time: 10 minutes	**Cooking Time:** 20 minutes	**Servings: 6 muffins**

Ingredients:

- ✓ 6 ounces ground almonds
- ✓ 1 teaspoon cinnamon
- ✓ ½ teaspoon baking powder
- ✓ 1 pinch sunflower seeds

Directions:

❖ Preheat oven to 350 degrees F. Line a muffin pan with paper muffin cups; set aside. Mix the almonds, cinnamon, baking powder, and sunflower seeds together and set aside. Take another bowl and whisk eggs, apple cider vinegar, applesauce, erythritol.

Ingredients:

- ✓ 1 whole egg
- ✓ 1 teaspoon apple cider vinegar
- ✓ 2 tablespoons erythritol
- ✓ 1/3 cup applesauce

❖ Add the mix to the dry ingredients and mix well until you have a smooth batter. Pour the batter into the mold and bake for 20 minutes. Once done, let them cool. Serve and enjoy!

233) MATCHA BOMB SUPREME

Preparation Time: 100 minutes	**Cooking Time:**	**Servings: 10**

Ingredients:

- ✓ 3/4 cup hemp seeds
- ✓ ½ cup coconut oil
- ✓ 2 tablespoons coconut almond butter
- ✓ 1 teaspoon Matcha powder

Directions:

❖ Take your blender/ food processor and add the hemp seeds, coconut oil, Matcha, vanilla extract and stevia.

Ingredients:

- ✓ 2 tablespoons vanilla bean extract
- ✓ ½ teaspoon mint extract
- ✓ Liquid stevia

❖ Blend until you have a nice batter and divide into silicone molds. Melt the coconut and almond butter and pour over top. Let the cups cool and enjoy!

234) PINEAPPLE HEARTY PUDDING

Preparation Time: 10 minutes	**Cooking Time:** 5 hours	**Servings: 4**

Ingredients:

- ✓ 1 teaspoon baking powder
- ✓ 1 cup coconut flour
- ✓ 3 tablespoons stevia
- ✓ 3 tablespoons avocado oil
- ✓ ½ cup coconut milk

Directions:

❖ Grease the Slow Cooker with oil. Take a bowl and mix the flour, stevia, baking powder, oil, milk, pecans, pineapple, lemon zest, pineapple juice and mix well.

Ingredients:

- ✓ ½ cup pecans, chopped
- ✓ ½ cup pineapple, chopped
- ✓ ½ cup lemon zest, grated
- ✓ 1 cup pineapple juice, natural

❖ Pour the mixture into the slow stove. Put the lid on and cook on LOW for 5 hours. Divide between bowls and serve. Enjoy!

235)	TASTY POACHED APPLES	
Preparation Time: 10 minutes	**Cooking Time**: 2 hours 30 minutes	**Servings**: 8

Ingredients:

- ✓ 6 apples, cored, peeled and sliced
- ✓ 1 cup apple juice, natural

Ingredients:

- ✓ 1 cup coconut sugar
- ✓ 1 tablespoon cinnamon powder

❖ Put the lid on and cook on HIGH for 4 hours. Serve cold and enjoy!

Directions:

❖ Grease the Slow Cooker with cooking spray. Add the apples, sugar, juice and cinnamon to the slow stove. Stir gently.

236)	HEART-WARMING CINNAMON RICE PUDDING	
Preparation Time: 10 minutes	**Cooking Time**: 5 hours	**Servings**: 4

Ingredients:

- ✓ 6 ½ cups water
- ✓ 1 cup coconut sugar
- ✓ 2 cups white rice

Ingredients:

- ✓ 2 cinnamon sticks
- ✓ ½ cup coconut, shredded

❖ Divide the pudding between dessert plates and enjoy!

Directions:

❖ Add the water, rice, sugar, cinnamon and coconut to your Slow Cooker. Stir gently. Put the lid on and cook on HIGH for 5 hours. Discard the cinnamon.

237)	SWEET ALMOND AND COCONUT FAT BOMBS	
Preparation Time: 10 minutes	**Cooking Time**: MOU4] Freezing Time: + 20 minutes	**Servings**: 6

Ingredients:

- ✓ ¼ cup melted coconut oil
- ✓ 9 ½ tablespoons almond butter
- ✓ 90 drops liquid stevia

Ingredients:

- ✓ 3 tablespoons cocoa
- ✓ 9 tablespoons melted almond butter sunflower seeds

❖ Chill for 20 minutes and take them out. Serve and enjoy!

Directions:

❖ Take a bowl and add all the ingredients listed. Mix them together well. Pour 2 tablespoons of the mixture into as many muffin molds as you want.

238)	THE MOST ELEGANT PARSLEY SOUFFLÉ EVER	
Preparation Time: 5 minutes	**Cooking Time:** 6 minutes	**Servings: 5**

Ingredients:

- ✓ 2 whole eggs
- ✓ 1 fresh red pepper, chopped

Ingredients:

- ✓ 2 tablespoons coconut cream
- ✓ 1 tablespoon fresh parsley, chopped
  Sunflower seeds to taste

Directions:

- ❖ Preheat oven to 390 degrees F. Butter almonds in 2 souffle dishes. Add ingredients to a blender and mix well. Divide the batter among the soufflé dishes and bake for 6 minutes. Serve and enjoy!

239)	EXUBERANT COCONUT CARAMEL	
Preparation Time: 20 minutes	**Cooking Time:** 2 hours	**Servings: 12**

Ingredients:

- ✓ ¼ cup coconut, shredded
- ✓ 2 cups coconut oil
- ✓ ½ cup coconut cream
- ✓ ¼ cup almonds, shredded

Ingredients:

- ✓ 1 teaspoon almond extract
- ✓ A pinch of sunflower seeds
- ✓ Stevia to taste

Directions:

- ❖ Take a large bowl and pour in the coconut cream and coconut oil. Whisk with an electric beater. Whisk until the mixture becomes smooth and glossy

- ❖ Add the cocoa powder slowly and mix well. Add the rest of the ingredients. Pour into a loaf pan lined with baking paper. Freeze until firm. Cut into squares and serve.

240)	PUMPKIN PUDDING WITH CHIA SEEDS EASY	
Preparation Time: 10-15 minutes	**Cooking Time:**	**Servings: 4**

Ingredients:

- ✓ 1 cup maple syrup
- ✓ 2 teaspoons pumpkin spice
- ✓ 1 cup pumpkin puree

Ingredients:

- ✓ 1 ¼ cup almond milk
- ✓ ½ cup chia seeds

Directions:

- ❖ Add all ingredients to a bowl and mix gently. Leave in the refrigerator overnight or at least 15 minutes. Add desired ingredients such as blueberries, almonds, etc. Serve and enjoy!

- ❖

241) DECISIVE LIME AND STRAWBERRY POPSICLE

Preparation Time: 2 hours	Cooking Time:	Servings: 4
✓ 1 tablespoon lime juice, fresh ✓ ¼ cup strawberries, hulled and sliced	✓ ¼ cup coconut almond milk, unsweetened and full-fat ✓ 2 teaspoons natural sweetener	
❖ Blend the listed ingredients in a blender until smooth. Pour mixture into popsicle molds and let cool for 2 hours. Serve and enjoy!		

242) COCONUT BREAD

Preparation Time: 15 minutes	Cooking Time: 40 minutes	Servings: 4
✓ 1 ½ tablespoons coconut flour ✓ ¼ teaspoon baking powder ✓ 1/8 teaspoon sunflower seeds	✓ 1 tablespoon coconut oil, melted ✓ 1 whole egg	
Directions: ❖ Preheat the oven to 350 degrees F. Add the coconut flour, baking powder, and sunflower seeds. Add the coconut oil, eggs and mix well until combined.	❖ Allow the batter to sit for a few minutes. Pour half of the batter onto the baking sheet. Spread to form a circle, repeat with remaining batter. Bake in the oven for 10 minutes. Once golden brown, let cool and serve. Enjoy!	

243) AUTHENTIC MEDJOOL DATE TRUFFLES

Preparation Time: 10-15 minutes	Cooking Time:	Servings: 4
✓ 2 tablespoons peanut oil ✓ ½ cup popcorn kernels ✓ 1/3 cup peanuts, chopped	✓ 1/3 cup almond and peanut butter ✓ ¼ cup wildflower honey	
Directions: ❖ Take a pot and add the popcorn kernels, peanut oil. Put it on medium heat and shake the pot gently until all the corn has popped.	❖ Take a saucepan and add the honey, simmer gently for 2-3 minutes. Add the almond and peanut butter and stir. Coat the popcorn with the mixture and enjoy!	

244) JUST A MINUTE THAT'S WORTH A MUFFIN

Preparation Time: 5 minutes	Cooking Time: 1 minute	Servings: 2
Ingredients: ✓ Coconut oil for greasing ✓ 2 teaspoons coconut flour ✓ 1 pinch baking soda	Ingredients: ✓ 1 pinch sunflower seeds ✓ 1 whole egg	
❖ Grease the ramekin with coconut oil and set aside. Add ingredients to a bowl and combine until there are no lumps. Pour the batter into the ramekin. Microwave for 1 minute on HIGH. Cut in half and serve. Enjoy!		

245) POACHED PEARS IN RED WINE

Preparation Time: 1 hour 35 minutes	**Cooking Time:**	**Servings: 4**

Ingredients:	Ingredients:
✓ 4 pears, peeled with stem intact ✓ 2 cups red wine ✓ 8 whole cloves ✓ 1 cinnamon stick	✓ ½ teaspoon vanilla extract ✓ 2 teaspoons sugar ✓ Creme fraiche for garnish

Directions:	
❖ In a saucepan over low heat, mix the red wine, cinnamon stick, cloves, vanilla extract and sugar and bring to a boil, stirring often until the sugar is dissolved. Add the pears, making sure they are submerged and boil for 15-20 minutes.	❖ Remove the pears to a plate and let the liquid simmer over medium heat for 15 minutes until reduced by half and syrupy. Remove from heat and let cool for 10 minutes. Drain to discard spices, allow to cool and pour over pears. Add the creme fraiche and serve.

246) SICILIAN GRANITA

Preparation Time: 5 minutes + freezing tme	**Cooking Time:**	**Servings: 4**

Ingredients:	Ingredients:
✓ 4 small oranges, chopped ✓ ½ teaspoon almond extract ✓ 2 tablespoons lemon juice	✓ 1 cup orange juice ✓ ¼ cup honey ✓ Fresh mint leaves for garnish

Directions:	
❖ In a food processor, blend the oranges, orange juice, honey, almond extract and lemon juice. Pulse until smooth. Pour into a dipping dish and freeze for 1 hour.	❖ Stir with a fork and freeze for another 30 minutes. Repeat a couple of times. Pour into dessert glasses and garnish with basil leaves. Serve immediately.

247) FRUIT CUPS WITH ORANGE JUICE

Preparation Time: 10 minutes	**Cooking Time:**	**Servings: 4**

Ingredients:	Ingredients:
✓ 1 cup orange juice ✓ ½ cup watermelon cubes ✓ 1 ½ cups grapes, cut in half ✓ 1 cup chopped melon	✓ ½ cup cherries, pitted and chopped ✓ 1 peach, chopped ✓ ½ teaspoon cinnamon powder

❖ Combine the watermelon cubes, grapes, cherries, cantaloupe and peach in a bowl. Add the orange juice and mix well. Distribute into dessert cups, sprinkle with cinnamon and serve cold.	

BIBLIOGRAPHY

FROM THE SAME AUTHOR

DASH DIET FOR HER Cookbook - More than 120 recipes for Women to reduce Cholesterol and Triglycerides! Start a Healthier lifestyle and Stop Hypertension with a Dietary Approach!

DASH DIET FOR BEGINNERS Cookbook - The Simplest and Quickest 120+ Dietary approach recipes to Stop Hypertension! Increase your heart health and reduce cholesterol and triglycerides with one of the healthiest diets overall!

DASH DIET FOR ONE Cookbook - More than Healthy 110 recipes to stop hypertension and reduce cholesterol! Stay Healthy and increase your body Wellness with the Best Dishes for One!

DASH DIET FOR HEALTHY KIDS' HEART Cookbook - More than 120 recipes for the health of your kids! Prevent Hypertension and Hearth Disease in your Children with one of the Best Diet Overall!

DASH DIET FOR TWO Cookbook - The Best 220+ Healthy Recipes to cook with your partner! Taste yourself and your love with many heart-health recipes for couple!

DASH DIET FOR HEALTHY COUPLE Cookbook - More than 220 Recipes for Two to reduce triglycerides and cholesterol! Delight Yourself and Your Partner with the Healthiest Dietary Approach Recipes!

DASH DIET FOR MUM & KIDS Cookbook - The Best 220+ Healthy and Quick Recipes to cook with your Kids! Delight yourself and your children and increase your heart health with the best Dietary Approach Recipes!

DASH DIET FOR START YOUR NEW HEALTHY LIFESTYLE Cookbook - More than 220 really health Recipes to Start by NOW the Dietary Approach. Increase your heart-health and reduce cholesterol and triglycerides with this Simple and Fantastic Diet!

DASH DIET FOR CHOLESTEROL CONTROL Cookbook - The Best 220+ Recipes to Reduce Bad Fat, Triglycerides, and Hypertension and Start to Have a New and Healthier Lifestyle!

CONCLUSION

Thanks for reading "The Dash Diet for Couple *Cookbook*"

Follow the right habits it is essential to have a healthy Lifestyle, and the Dash diet is the best solution!

I hope you liked this Cookbook and I wish you to achieve all your goals!

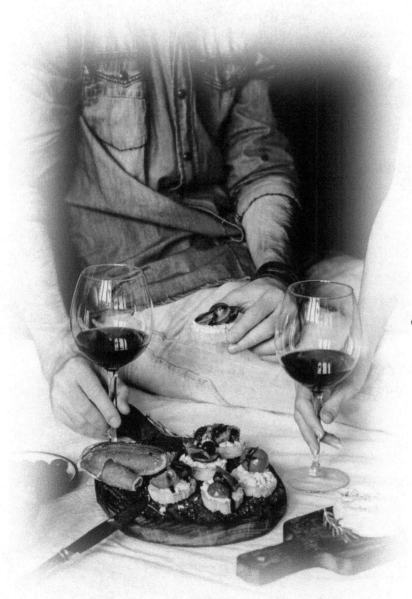

Michelle Sandler